Sex, Health and Nutrition

Dr Robert L. Erdmann is in private practice at Medabolics Limited, 14 Mount Pleasant Road, Tunbridge Wells, England, TN1 1QU. Telephone: 0892 542609.

Meirion Jones is a public relations consultant and health writer. He co-authored *Fats, Nutrition and Health* with Robert Erdmann.

Sex, Health and Nutrition

Robert Erdmann, Ph.D.
and Meirion Jones

Thorsons
An Imprint of HarperCollins*Publishers*

Thorsons
An Imprint of HarperCollins*Publishers*
77–85 Fulham Palace Road,
Hammersmith, London W6 8JB

Published by Thorsons 1992
1 3 5 7 9 10 8 6 4 2

A catalogue record for this book
is available from the British Library

ISBN 0 7225 2230 4

Typeset by Harper Phototypesetters Limited,
Northampton, England
Printed in Great Britain by
Mackays of Chatham, Kent

Contents

Preface

First the Dark Ages . . .

The late 1940s and early 1950s found me on the threshold of adulthood and, in common with most young people, I was eager to learn about sex. It's very difficult now, in the aftermath of the permissive explosion of the sixties and seventies, to imagine the level of ignorance, and perhaps even fear, of sex at that time. Except for an endless but unenlightening round of smutty jokes and stories, sex was never openly discussed. It was simply not considered to be an acceptable social or educational topic. Even questions of a sexual nature to parents were stonewalled by embarrassing silences. Books such as *The Kama Sutra*, Henry Miller's *The Tropic of Cancer* and *The Tropic of Capricorn* and D. H. Lawrence's *Lady Chatterley's Lover* were on the banned book list.

Consequently, in this atmosphere of suppressed knowledge, the more unacceptable sex seemed to be as a topic of interest, the more interested I became in it. Anything of the slightest relevance was seized upon like crusts to a starving man: straightforward biological information gleaned from musty text books, 'how to' techniques passed down from the older brothers of my friends, even documentary photographs of naked tribespeople torn from copies of *The National Geographic Magazine*.

All this bred a level of knowledge that was barely more than superstition. Not surprisingly in that climate, myths were taken as fact. Masturbation, for example, was commonly believed to cause mental illness and physical weakness. When a report was published – the Kinsey survey on *Sexual Behavior in the Human Male* – showing how common masturbation was, many people saw it as the cause of the illogical and crazy behaviour of the young. The dark ages indeed.

. . . Then the Enlightenment

Finally, I went away to college, armed with a formidable arsenal of sexual jokes and stories and an insatiable appetite for discovery. College, to my delight, proved to be a great place to extend my knowledge. It was full of young men and women living away from home, free for the first time from direct parental supervision.

My course – majoring in psychology and minoring in sociology – allowed me to pursue my main interest with a passion and dedication unequalled by most of my contemporaries. Everything I studied I related to sex. This was easy with subjects such as psychology, sociology, romantic literature, and physiology, but regardless of the subject – be it chemistry, microbiology, even military science and statistics – I twisted the material until I made the sexual connection. Not easily embarrassed, I would brazenly ask every tutor, male or female, questions that probed the depth of their knowledge, developing in the process an almost encyclopaedic store of technical information. My friends said jokingly but with good cause that I had sperm for brain cells.

By the end of the course it seemed to me that there was a terrific need for accurate sexual information and counselling. Morals were expected to control sexual behaviour, but from what I'd seen and experienced it was the hormones that won out every time. The conflict between social customs and sexual desires, coupled with widespread ignorance, meant that there were a lot of unhappy and frustrated people about.

The Modern Age

And now, a supposed sexual revolution later, here we are in the present: a time when sex is openly discussed, when sex before marriage is the norm rather than the exception, when there are numerous outlets for expressing sexual difficulties and hang-ups, when sex is looked upon and accepted as a fulfilling recreation. Perhaps in our post-AIDS society the idea of free sex has taken a battering, but even the most ardent campaigners will never be able to stuff it back into the cupboard from whence it sprang.

Yet problems remain. Frigidity, impotence, premature ejaculation, and an inability to orgasm are widespread difficulties, causing anguish, strained relationships, and uncertainty. It is generally accepted that such problems have emotional and psychological causes. In contrast, I believe that their roots lie not solely in psychological imbalances but also in nutritional ones. Everyone knows how strongly food influences both behaviour and physical performance. Alcohol alters your ability to think and act, coffee makes you more alert and gives you energy. These are crude examples well known by everyone. Only now are we discovering the subtle ways in which all food and water influence every aspect of our health and behaviour. Quite simply, bad food or inadequate nourishment causes illness and disability. On the other hand, give the body all the nutrients it needs to perform, to carry out its millions of complex chemical functions, and its resistance to disease will grow, energy levels and strength will increase and, as a welcome consequence, good, fulfilling sex will be an added benefit.

This is quite a sweeping claim. However, my work as a nutritionist has led me to treat many people suffering from sexual disability, and time and time again I've seen patients' sexual problems disappear simply by modifying their diets and supplementing them with special nutrients. The body is, after all, made from food, water, and air. Once in the body these nutrients are used in complex ways but, none the less, it is they that provide the raw materials for the hormones, organs, muscles, brain chemicals, and energy we need for sex. Improve the quality of the food you eat, therefore, and your sex life will benefit. This applies not just to those experiencing difficulties, but also to people whose sex lives are already satisfactory and are looking to make them even better.

Of course, this isn't always as easy as it sounds, which is why Meirion and I have written this together. It explains what nutrients the body needs for good sex, how they are used, where to obtain them – from dietary sources as well as food supplements – and the benefits you can expect to reap. I've greatly enjoyed the research involved in this book, especially as it brings together two of my greatest interests – sex and nutrition – and I hope you enjoy it, and the consequences of following its advice, too. Happy reading.

Robert Erdmann
January 1992

Part 1
Introduction

Chapter 1
Sense and Sexuality

Emily, a 54-year-old widow, has recently experienced a sexual revelation. Her husband, a lawyer, died of heart attack when she was 45 and for the last nine years she has lived alone, solitary and celibate. The reason for this is not a lack of suitors. She was, and remains, a strikingly handsome woman. She is intelligent, quick-witted, and a successful career-woman in her own right, having risen to a senior post in the civil service before her retirement. However, in the years following her bereavement, despite an acknowledged need for love and companionship, she candidly describes how she became 'formidably unapproachable'.

'It was as if my husband's death was the trigger for character changes – a classic Jekyll and Hyde transformation drawn out painfully over several years,' she says. 'I became increasingly intolerant and short-tempered and wilfully obstructive. I drove men away.'

Those few relationships she did strike up were short-lived. 'My husband and I had enjoyed a fairly happy sex life. It was nothing extravagant but it was important to both of us. But with the men I did attempt to sleep with afterwards – sensitive, understanding men – sex became a hideous experience. It was painful, dry, and passionless.' Emily interpreted the emotional and physical difficulties as signs that she was entering her menopause and, to compensate, she diverted her attention and energies into her work, perhaps as a way of shielding herself from the physical changes. Submerging herself in her job, her personal life was neglected and she passed into retirement without a partner.

Last she she visited America to spend some time with her daughter and son-in-law. There she met, was courted by, and fell in love with Emmet, a 62-year-old associate at her daughter's law firm. 'He is in his mid-sixties but he has the vitality and enthusiasm for life I would have associated with someone 30 years younger. He plays racquetball, swims, parties, and', she says dropping her voice, 'he has a large sexual appetite. To cut a long story short, I didn't know what to do. I wanted to be with him, to share his desires with him, but for the past nine years or so I'd considered myself physically incapable of sex. Frankly I was terrified at the prospect of sleeping with him but also terrified by the thought I might lose him.'

Finally, they just talked. 'I didn't know how he'd react, but what I didn't expect was for him to say in so many words: "Goddamnit, we're going to beat this thing." Emmet had friends in a local health-food store who in turn put us in contact with a nutritional counsellor – which, when I heard it mentioned, I thought was someone who gave advice to overeaters.' The counsellor turned out to be an expert on the way that nutritional supplements – such as vitamins and minerals – can be used to improve the healthy workings of the body. During a couple of consultations she devised a programme of supplementation for Emily which she was to follow religiously.

'I'm not exactly clear how these supplements managed to do what they did; whatever the technicalities are, they actually seemed to reverse many of the effects of the menopause. I became more relaxed about myself, felt confident about experiencing and returning Emmet's desire for me. I started menstruating again. I even had an orgasm.' As far as Emily's sex life is concerned, she claims that the supplements help give her an excitement and sense of discovery that she cannot remember having experienced before.

In contrast, excitement and discovery were the last words that Colin, a television producer, would have used to describe his sex life.

'It's not that I didn't look forward to sex, I did. I love Heike, my wife, dearly. Yet, when it came to the act, it was as if I was a distant, disinterested observer. I felt detached and unenthused. It was impossible to get a proper erection, no matter how much foreplay we tried. On the few occasions I was able to penetrate I felt no desire and my penis would quickly go flaccid.'

They went to their doctor who in turn sent them to a marriage guidance counsellor. The consensus was that Colin's difficulties were largely a state of mind. Since he wasn't suffering from any sort of disease that may have caused the problem – such as diabetes – it was felt to be his attitude that was at fault. They were given touch exercises and routines to follow to reawaken his interest, but all to no effect.

Happily, the marriage guidance counsellor also suggested that Colin visit a nutritional therapist. He did so and at the end of his visit was handed a list of supplements to take. ('Things I'd never heard of – amino acids, essential fatty acids – as well as a load of vitamins and minerals.') Very quickly, the supplements started to take effect. 'I had more energy, not just in bed but everywhere. Heike was very desirable again and I now find myself sometimes almost intoxicated by her sex. I'm now thinking of cutting down a bit since they've had such a dramatic effect.'

This book is called *Sex, Nutrition and Health*. It's based around a very simple premise: namely, for better or for worse, the food that we eat can alter the quality of our sex lives. Good food – rich in the vital nutrients of life – deepens and prolongs the experience of sex, making us more sensitive, more receptive, more desirable, and more energetic. Bad food – refined, polluted and unadulterated – has the opposite effect. In this book we'll explain why.

Now, surely, a note of scepticism is called for here. After all, the idea of reversing Emily's metabolic clock or alleviating what would seem to be a problem with Colin's attitude of mind simply by taking a selection of dietary supplements does seem a bit far-fetched. But is it really? Or are we only conditioned to think of these problems as irreversible or unalterable, to shrug our shoulders and accept that nature must take its course and that there is nothing we can do to change it. If so, it is surely this conditioning that makes us accept that the menopause advances like an inexorable tide, and makes us perceive impotence or frigidity or premature ejaculation as arbitrary products of an unstable imagination, problems to be alleviated, if at all, by some nebulous bout of positive thinking.

This book shows you how to take such attitudes by the scruff of the neck, shove them aside, and start doing something positive and creative about your sex life. It achieves this primarily by showing you the sorts of nutrients available for helping to improve your sexual performance, nutrients that affect you on an emotional level as well as a physical one. It explains how to construct special diets rich in the relevant nutrients, and how carefully targeted dietary supplements can enhance and energise your life in a way you might never have imagined. It also contains the case histories of individuals who have successfully used the methods explained in this book to effect change in their own lives; only their names have been changed. Before plunging into the heart of the book, though, it is important to understand just how food is able to affect us in this way. This means a brief, and simple, introduction to the metabolic processes of your body. So let's take a short detour away from all this talk about sex, and travel instead deep down into the innermost workings of the body.

The Sex in your Food

Look closely at your skin, at the familiar wrinkles and hairs, the occasional moles, and the light-brown tan. Look closer, much closer, and this view will be transformed into an ocean of million upon million of cells oscillating with chemical and electromagnetic energy. These cells make up the skin, bone, hair, muscles, organs, glands, and fats as well as blood, hormones, enzymes, and other fluids of your body. Furthermore, each one of these uncountable millions is unique to your body and your special bodily needs. They are needed for growth and regeneration, to ward off illness, and repair damage, and because these are tremendous demands their mortality rate is high. Accepting this, the next question is how do we ensure a constant supply of replacements for the dead and exhausted cells?

The obvious answer is, of course, we obtain them from the

food that we eat and drink, and, less obviously, from the air that we breathe. But how do the roast chicken, carrots, peas, potatoes, and gravy you had for lunch become the highly specialised cells of the body? They don't. No more than the parts of, say, a decommissioned battleship – gun turrets, anchors, and compass – would be used directly to build a locomotive train. However, in the same way that all the reusable materials would be stripped from their battleship at the breaker's yard and melted or ground down into their simplest components before being refashioned into totally new shapes for the train, so is the food we eat reworked to form the body's cells.

Once in the stomach and gut, powerful acids and enzymes tear the food apart, breaking it down into its individual cells and then even further into the constituent nutrient molecules that make the cells up. The flesh of the chicken, for example, is broken up into individual protein molecules and these molecules are then separated into their building blocks, a group of substances known as amino acids. If food that was not fully digested was absorbed into the body it would have an effect similar to what happens when a transplanted organ is rejected by the host body: a violent response resembling a life-threatening allergy. The digestion process, therefore, needs to be ruthlessly thorough.

Once the food has been split bit by bit into its simplest possible constituents it is absorbed through the intestine wall and passed into the blood stream. Even then different stretches of the bowel are modified to absorb different classes of nutrient such as amino acid, vitamin, mineral, carbohydrate, or fat so that they enter the body in selected groupings to make distribution easier. These tiny nutrients are now ready to be reconstructed as the complex and specialised cells that we have just looked at. What next?

The Body Politic

It would be no exaggeration to say that in many ways the body's functions often mirror those of an entire country. The body's brain, for example, is the centre for a disproportionately high level of energy and metabolic activity in the same way that a country's capital city attracts a high proportion of the populace, capital, investment, and growth. Like this capital city, the brain governs the entire body by sending out edicts in the form of electrical nerve transmissions or messenger chemicals. The motorways of the body are the circulatory system. Teeming with more 'vehicles' than the bumper-to-bumper traffic of the Monday morning rush hour, the arteries ferry cargoes of vital nutrients wherever they are needed in the body.

If you consider how many different activities occur each day in a country, the messages, conversations, building projects, demolition sites, journeys, and shopping expeditions, as well as the amount of cargo carried and waste created, you start to get an inkling of how much goes on in the body. So how do the raw materials – the nutrients that were once your Sunday lunch – fit into this, and more importantly, how do they relate to sex? The answer is by means of the metabolic pathways. You'll be hearing a lot about these in the pages to come.

The Whirlpool of Creation

The metabolic pathways are transformation processes with many stages in which the individual raw-material nutrients are brought together to form large and more complicated molecules. The end products of these transformations can then be put to use for whatever specific body task they have been created.

Metabolic pathways are created by the secretion of different sorts of hormones. These are messenger chemicals, the body's despatch riders. They carry orders from the brain, ensuring functions such as the body's ability to grow, repair, prepare for action, respond to stress, combat infection, and reproduce are carried out. Hormones play a key role in our story and they'll be cropping up many times. Depending on what sort of end products need to be created from the raw materials, the hormones can order another set of important chemicals, called enzymes, to start fusing the separate nutrients together. This is accomplished by following special nucleic acid blueprints known as DNA and RNA which contain all the information on which nutrient should be used where. Raw materials are bonded to each other according to the template of these nucleic acids. Each bonding represents a separate stage of the metabolic pathway. This process can become so complex that for some pathways many hundreds of nutrients might be involved at various stages of creation.

The Components of Life

Understanding how many of these nutrients work in the body is central to full sexual performance, emotionally and physically. We'll be meeting these nutrients frequently in the pages to come, and you'll learn how to exploit their key roles in the metabolic pathways to help enhance and fulfill your expectations and experiences of good sex. Because of this, a few brief introductions are in order. Very simply, there are five major groupings of nutrients: amino acids, essential fatty acids, carbohydrate, vitamins, and minerals.

Of these five, the first two, amino acids and essential fatty acids, make up what is known as the body's substrate. This means that they form the underlying physical structures of every substance in the body. Amino acids, for example, are the proverbial building blocks of protein. A core of 22 separate aminos can be linked in the metabolic pathways to create at least 50,000 different forms of protein. Some of these are enzymes for breaking down, as with digestion, or for bonding together. Others are used as hormones in such functions as neurotransmitters (the body's brain-message chemicals, which we'll be seeing a lot of). Still others make up the helix-shaped scaffolding of fibrous protein: while most people realise that the skin is made largely from protein, they don't know that the same is true of bone, into which is built the metabolic concrete of calcium phosphate.

Essential fatty acids are less well known than the amino acids but are equally important. Like amino acids, they and their derivatives serve a variety of functions from acting as hormones and other regulatory molecules to forming the basic foundations of the body's structure. They form the building blocks of triglycerides and phosphatides, substances which, because of their insolubility in water, form the surface of every cell wall in the body. Few people think of fat as anything other than the reason for not eating too many cream cakes but, as we'll see, they are as important as protein.

As for the remaining food groups, vitamins and minerals make up what are known as the co-factors. They help the substrate chemicals to form new structures in the metabolic pathways; vitamin C, for example, is the essential bonding component of the structural protein collagen. The co-factors also play important roles in their own right. They regulate the body's pH (acid) balance, maintain its electrical potential (the body is, after all, an electromagnetic organism), and keep the water retention balanced between inside the cell and out.

Finally, the last of the group is carbohydrate, a food that provides us with the primary source of energy for all the metabolic reactions to take place.

As we've said, the above forms the briefest of introductions and in the course of the book we'll get to know these nutrients much more intimately. For now, let's see how they interact in practice. To take one example, let's watch what happens to an amino acid called phenylalanine. Phenylalanine sits at the start of a metabolic pathway which, due to the action of various enzymes, sees the creation of several important hormones including l-dopa, a chemical used to calm nerve activity; adrenalin, the one hormone that we've probably all heard of and the one responsible for our ability to withstand and respond to stress; alpha endorphins, the body's natural painkillers, produced in times of stress; and phenylethylamine (PEA), a so-called 'love chemical' thought to be responsible for arousing strong feelings of attraction and desire.

The nutrient co-factors needed to effect this stage-by-stage conversion include magnesium, phosphorus, copper, vitamin C, numerous B vitamins, and three different enzymes. And don't forget, the enzymes are themselves the products of other metabolic pathways.

Of course, this isn't the only use for phenylalanine. As an amino acid it is an essential component in the manufacture of proteins. Together with its 21 sibling aminos it is strung together in differing combinations to create a wide assortment of different protein structures: keratin for hair, myosin for muscles, and collagen for skin are just three examples. Each of these requires the active involvement of vitamins, minerals, and essential fatty acids. As the cell structures created by metabolic pathways become exhausted, they are broken apart by enzymes, some material salvaged, some burnt to release energy, and the rest excreted – again, key roles performed by the metabolic pathways.

Metabolic pathways and the nutrients that ply them are a cyclical, self-regenerating, interrelated series of chemical reactions. Sooner or later, one nutrient having been brought into a pathway by the action of an enzyme will reach a stage where, as a component of another enzyme, it will itself participate in the creation of the first enzyme that reacted with it. Confusing? This ability to recreate itself is the enigma of life. Scientists have mapped out hundred upon hundred of these metabolic pathways and they resemble nothing so much as a huge whirlpool seen from above. The chemical products of the pathways look like the whirlpool's currents, forced out from the centre of the swirling vortex and breaking into ever more intricate waves and eddies before being sucked back towards the centre to create other new currents.

It is worth making one point crystal clear. Metabolic pathways are responsible for everything. Not only do they form our muscles, but they create the chemicals needed to release the energy needed to move them. Not only do they manufacture the brain cells, but they create the chemicals which carry the brain messages and which control our behaviour. Metabolic pathways, therefore, are the source of wellbeing for the mind and the body. And, not coincidentally, sex just happens to be the balance between the mind and the body. To see how this links up, let's now look at the metabolic actions involved in sex, each of which, don't forget, is the result of a metabolic pathway. This will become clearer later.

Spark to Ignition

Sex begins as a subtle psychological flicker and ends in a physical act that blots out thought. From beginning to end, though, it is under the control of the body's glands and hormones. Typically, sexual arousal begins with one of the five senses responding to stimulation. It might be the sight of an attractive person, or their scent (the sense of smell is a particularly strong arousal trigger). It may be their voice, not only its sound but what is said. More intimately, it may be the way they taste, or the way they touch.

Most likely, it is a combination of these experiences which causes the first inklings of sexual arousal: a metabolic 'amber alert' in a gland called the hypothalamus situated just above the mid-brain. The alert triggers other glands into commencing the process of arousal, both emotional and physical. The first to respond is the medulla, a section of the brain, which orders the lungs to breathe more quickly and the heart to beat more rapidly. This provides more food, and more oxygen in which to burn it to release energy. Simultaneously, the alert spreads elsewhere and the limbic system begins to secrete the neurotransmitter (brain chemical) phenylethylamine or PEA. It is PEA which shifts the arousal up a gear, introducing powerful emotions such as love and desire as well as leading to a narrower mental focus.

It is at about this time that the arousal baton is passed from the emotional sphere to the physical. Physical contact and stimulation between the partners, together with the release of two neurotransmitter hormones, adrenalin and acetylcholine, leads to the erection of penis and clitoris. These hormones trigger the sympathetic nervous system, or fight-or-flight response. This causes blood to be diverted from non-essential functions such as digestion. Instead, the blood flows into the dilating arterial vessels of the sex organs and is prevented from leaving by the constriction of the outflowing veins. The result is an inflating and hardening of the tissue. The action of these two hormones in women also leads to the secretion of mucus inside the vagina, while in men it causes the cowper glands to secrete lubricating fluid. Once penetration occurs these lubricants ease the contact between penis and vaginal wall, the absence of friction in turn allowing a rhythmic massaging action.

This massage action causes the release of oxytocin, a hormone that triggers involuntary vibrations of the pelvis, further intensifying the response. Meanwhile, fat-derived chemicals called prostaglandins are causing the cervix to shudder and convulse. At the same time the body is secreting morphine-like chemicals called endorphins to block any sensations not relevant to the immediate sexual response. The clichés found in romantic novels about being swept away, floating on a sea of love, or drugged with desire are, from a biochemical point of view, quite accurate.

Finally, when the intensity of the massage is sufficient, orgasm occurs. This is an involuntary reflex caused by the release of a substance called histamine from cells in the head of the penis and in the clitoris. Semen from the man's prostate gland and seminal vesicles situated beneath his bladder is ejected in a series of muscle spasms. This acts as a neural circuit breaker and hormonal activity ceases.

This is what happens when sex goes right. However, this book is partly about showing how you can rectify things when they go wrong. What does go wrong and why is what we'll look at next.

Out of Balance

Nowadays farming is, on the whole, a precise, scientific business. Crops are reared in huge, hedgeless fields and harvested to suit the just-in-time distribution cycles of the supermarkets. To grow these crops quickly, and to produce consistently shaped specimens that look pleasantly plump, phosphate and nitrate fertilisers are used intensively. These fertilisers, though, interfere with the vegetables' absorption of important minerals, especially trace elements such as zinc and copper (remember zinc, it will figure very strongly in later chapters on sexual performance). Acid rain – produced from the nitrous oxide and sulphur dioxide clouds that billow like brimstone from our power stations – also does its fair share of damage. Falling onto the soil as sulphuric and nitric acid it prevents the crops from absorbing large quantities of most minerals.

A word on the aforementioned just-in-time distribution cycles of the supermarkets. These are superbly organised ways of ensuring that supply meets demand. High-powered, fourth-generation, computer mainframe-linked information systems present detailed information on consumer buying trends in the form of vivid, colourful graphics. Sitting at his computer terminal, a purchasing accountant notices a buying trend develop on a particular crop. He brushes the 'purchase' symbol on his touch-sensitive infra-red screen sending an order to buy heavily on that crop. A farmer receives a phone call. 'Harvest now!' says a voice. It doesn't matter that his crop isn't yet ripe, that it should be given time to mature, to absorb more vital minerals and vitamins. Finally, the denuded crop arrives in the shops, the anticipated customer demand materialises, and shoppers go home with an unripe product, short of nutrition.

OK, so you buy organic when you can, which isn't as often or as thoroughly as you'd like considering supply outstrips demand hundreds to one. What about meat? Well, many pigs are fed on a growth hormone called sulphidimine. Perfectly healthy says MAFF. Not so says the FDA; we are withdrawing its licence forthwith as a potential carcinogen. The fact is, no one really knows how widespread and profound are the effects of growth hormones on the human body, but these hormones are injected as a matter of course into cows and pigs.

However, the FDA doesn't get away that lightly. MAFF is currently testing bovine somatotrophin (BST), a hormone that increases milk yields in dairy cows. No one knows what the long-term effects of this hormone are. Yet the ministry won't even reveal which herds are being used and where. This hormone has already been provisionally accepted in the US despite the fact that the FDA was forced to sack one of its most senior and trusted advisers, Richard Burroughs, for expressing safety concerns over the use of BST. By giving a green light to the hormone, Burroughs felt that the FDA contravened its own safety rules. It is hard to imagine such laxity being applied to the testing and approval of nutritional supplements.

Antibiotics are another cause of anxiety. This 'medicine', which is known to kill off the body's own intestinal flora and weaken its immune system is used widely on both pigs and cows. Chicken? All but the genuinely free-range varieties are fed on an outrageous slurry of low-value nutrients: feathers, ground beaks, you name it. Factory-farmed chicken doesn't just lack taste, it lacks the nutrient quality of an animal reared in a natural foraging environment.

As for much of the processed food available in the shops, this is really a continuation of the denuding started by intensive farming. Yet how many people can be bothered to cook with fresh foods every night? We rely on processed, packaged foods to make our lives more convenient. Furthermore, we are all prey to the sophisticated marketing techniques of food companies anxious to dispell any worry over food quality. A recent report by the supposedly independent British Dental Health Foundation into the causes of tooth decay, for example, didn't once mention sugar as a probable culprit; not surprising when you realise that the sugar industry's lobbying arm, the Sugar Bureau, is a member of the foundation and brought immense pressure to bear on the form of the final report. Yes, processed food is convenient. Yet there is an impressive amount of literature to indicate that we are also short-changing our health in using it.

Stepping Back

We realise that much of what we are saying will sound Luddite, blaming computers and food-processing techniques and state-of-the-art fertilisers and probably well-meaning government ministries for the state of our food. However, we are not espousing a return to some agricultural paradise of organic smallholding. It never existed and, if it were to, would be totally unable to meet the food demands of the country. What would be wonderful to see, though, would be all this technological efficiency and government zeal turned to encouraging the nourishment and growth of truly large-scale organic farming. We would like to see responsible and open education programmes enlightening people on the true value of the food they buy in the shops – with the support of the producers. As it is, properly healthy, balanced diets are prohibitively expensive for a large selection of the populace (the health education authority estimates that it is actually beyond the reach of many people on a low income), and impractical for many others.

What we have looked at so far is the potentially disastrous quality of our food. This book is largely about raising that quality and, in turn, raising the quality of your life as a whole and your sex life in particular. Before we go any further, though, it's worth bearing in mind that achieving this aim can be hard work. We don't claim to be able to present you with a sex-improving capsule, or a potent menu of aphrodisiac food to stimulate you. All we can do is show you how to exploit ordinary everyday nutrition, which should be ours by right, to enhance your sexuality, physically and emotionally.

Summary

Sex is a complex biochemical balance of emotional and physical responses. These responses need adequate supplies of numerous chemicals and these are made in the body's metabolic pathways from the raw materials contained in the food we eat. Although our society is food rich, many factors prevent us from obtaining the quality of food necessary for supplying the metabolic pathways.

Chapter 2
Sexual Problems are not All in the Mind

A close friend of ours, Peter, is a biochemist in the chemicals subsidiary of one of the world's largest oil companies. He works as part of a research team and his job is to create new chemical compounds and then develop applications for them. Once patented, these chemicals will be marketed for use in one or more of a diverse range of applications: as a colouring or flavouring agent in food, for example; as an acidity regulator or preservative; as a means of improving the non-drip qualities of paint; and even as a new drug to aid blood-clotting or to improve short-term memory. Peter's knowledge of biochemistry is immense. In the course of a dinner party conversation or bar-room chat terms such as 'arachidonic cascade' and 'lipid peroxidation' trip off his tongue with the ease and enthusiasm of a devoted sports fan recalling who knocked in the winning putt in the 1973 Ryder Cup golf tournament. In short, he knows the metabolic pathways inside out.

When we told him we were going to write a book on the way in which sexual performance can be enhanced by supplementing the metabolic pathways with nutrients, he was flabbergasted. 'You're joking,' he said. 'What can you say? What are you going to write about? Nutrition has nothing at all to do with sex. Sexual problems are all psychological.'

His incredulity illustrates a curious kind of doublethink typical of orthodox scientists and doctors. Look at it. They are educated in an atmosphere of scientific rigour. They are taught that behind today's knowledge lie theories which, before being accepted as fact, must be subjected to stringent analysis and testing. Double-blind tests on large numbers of subjects, exhaustive processing of the results, and statistically significant conclusions are the currency of their work. New discoveries on the secrets of metabolism – on the creation of enzymes, perhaps, or the release of energy and the effects of different nutrients on physical performance – are questioned exhaustively, papers published, and disagreements about their significance aired.

The medical profession prides itself on this *modus operandi*. And rightly so. Yet, like any rigid system for looking at and understanding the body, it does have its shortcomings. One of these is the faintly disturbing way in which the human body and all its functions are seen as nothing more than a complicated machine, the whole dazzling phenomenon of life viewed in terms of abstruse chemical formulas, such as Peter's arachidonic cascades and lipid peroxides. It is this sort of approach that sees the thinking and reasoning processes of man – his ability to evolve moral principles and philosophical notions of reality – as nothing more than a biochemical telephone exchange, with its billions of neurons passing electrical impulses to each other via neurotransmitters to create neural memory circuits. A concept as difficult, and as precious, as the mind is defined as a mechanism, one whose individual components are no more than separate, identifiable chemicals.

This model of human beings is very useful when it comes to analysing the need for nutrients. After all, if the body is a mechanism that functions effectively thanks to its raw material chemicals, then it follows that a shortage of chemical nutrients will prevent it from functioning properly, resulting in such deficiency diseases as beriberi, pellagra, scurvy, anaemia, and so on, not to mention illnesses caused by the wrong sort of food such as cardiovascular disease and obesity. All this the medical and scientific community asserts, our biochemist friend included. This is where the doublethink comes in.

If we take their own logic at face value and, by using their own way of looking at the body, apply these same principles to invoke a direct connection between nutrition and sex, many of these eminent men and women of science will deafen you with their protests. 'No, no,' they will cry. 'Sexual problems are psychological problems.' In other words, it's a problem of the mind, not the body. But wait a minute. Just where does the mechanistic model of the body as a machine to be explored and mapped out hand over to this nebulous, unquantifiable

phantom known as the mind? When does a physical problem
become a psychological problem? Where is the line drawn? AS
FAR AS THIS BOOK IS CONCERNED, THERE IS NO LINE!
Let us explain why.

Psychology refers to a so-called 'state of mind'. This state of
mind – its level of contentment, tranquillity, anxiety, stress,
fear, excitement, learning, inquisitiveness – is, according to
what has been proven by science, produced by billions of
neural interconnections which are, in turn, created by
neurotransmitters. The neurotransmitters themselves are
chemical compounds produced by raw materials obtained
from our diet. If neurotransmitters affect human psychology
and diet affects neurotransmitters, then diet has a bearing on
psychology, and in particular the psychology of sex. QED.

We're not saying that all mental problems can be traced
directly to diet. Far from it. What we are saying is that a
connection exists. As far as we are concerned, and as the work
of numerous nutritionists in treating sexual problems shows,
this connection is as irrefutable as the existence of the Golden
Gate Bridge. And as the bridge links one piece of land with
another, so this book aims to link a good diet with good sex. To
say, as Peter did, that sexual difficulties are psychological in
origin as if that were the end of the matter rather than the start
seems to be a failure not only of imagination but of belief in the
very tenets of his profession. He seems willing to go so far in
his assertion that man is only a biochemical machine but no
further.

A recent article in a British newspaper renowned for its
enlightened attitude towards alternative health mirrors this
very attitude. The article discusses the degree to which myalgic
encephalomyelitis (otherwise known as ME or post-viral
syndrome) is a psychosomatic illness. Bearing in mind that
many of its symptoms are similar to depression, some doctors
feel that it is at least partly a psychological problem. Yet
describing it as psychological alienates many of the sufferers.
It makes them feel they are mentally unstable. In fact, as we will
see in chapter 3, some causes of depression are discernibly
physical in origin. Many cases have been treated successfully
with amino acid supplements and other nutritional aids.
In fact the article even revealed that medicines based on
the amino acid tryptophan – precursor of the inhibitory
neurotransmitter, serotonin – can help to relieve symptoms by

treating depression. For the writer, this seemed to confirm that their problems were psychological. Yet surely a lack of the relevant depression-fighting neurotransmitters is first and foremost a physical problem.

No doubt Peter will continue to disagree with us. This schism between the mental and the physical perception of metabolism is set to stay with us for a long time yet. It is worth remembering, though, that this curious doublethink exists. Remind yourself of it if you ever find yourself with a sexual problem being told by your doctor that it's 'purely psychological'. Make him uncomfortable, ask him exactly what he means.

Sex: the Metabolic Merry-Go-Round

So how does nutrition alter sexual performance. What areas of this 'psychological' activity do we have the knowledge to affect? In the following chapters we'll see how fatty acids, amino acids, vitamins, minerals, herbal remedies, and carefully chosen diets can be applied to the relevant metabolic pathways to bring about positive changes to your sexuality. One important point that you should always bear in mind, though, is that whatever can be achieved with nutritional supplementation is attained by carefully blending the supplements so that they assist each other. By using a blend of nutrients you strengthen the metabolic pathways as a whole, rather than just one area.

To illustrate the point, let's take the rest of this chapter to look at some of the sex nutrients at work, complementing each other. Each nutrient, and its effects, will be examined in greater depth later.

To Come or not Come

For many men premature ejaculation is a frustrating, unsatisfying, and often humiliating experience. And, par for the course, all too often it is summarily dismissed with the assurance that it's just a state of mind, that in time everything will turn out all right. (Another friend who suffered from this problem was told by his doctor, 'Don't worry, old chap, it'll all come out in the wash'; a less appropriate choice of words is hard to imagine.)

There is a large body of research that suggests that ejaculation for the male and orgasm for both sexes are affected by a substance called histamine. Circulating in the blood and stored in many cells of the body, histamine participates in a number of important chemical reactions including the body's immune response to infection and injury. Histamine causes the redness, swelling, and inflammation of skin tissue around wounds or as a response to allergy. It also causes chill sensations, shivering, sneezing, hives, migraine, and skin flushing. Interestingly, all these responses in some degree are common to the sex response.

As the trigger of orgasm, histamine is concentrated in what are called mast cells. These are found in the glans penis of the male and clitoris of the female. When sexual stimulation reaches its peak, the histamine bursts from these cells and orgasm occurs. Higher than average levels of histamine have been related to an early release from the mast cells and consequently lead to premature ejaculation. Conversely, the inability to ejaculate or achieve orgasm, called rather flippantly frigidity, has been associated with below average levels of histamine.

Histamine is also used by the body to stimulate the production of stomach acid, a function which, as we shall see in chapter 3, is important for overall health and wellbeing. Finally, the brain uses it as a neuro-inhibitor, lowering the frequency of the frantic beta brain waves and thereby helping to combat anxiety. Histamine is an important nutritional component of the sex response and, by devoting an entire chapter to it (chapter 6), we'll show you what you can do to regulate its levels in your body.

Carrying the Sex Message

Histamine, though, isn't the only substance to affect the brain's sex response. We've already seen how important many neurotransmitters are for sustaining emotional balance and wellbeing. There is considerable evidence to show that certain neurotransmitters have an even more direct effect on sexual response.

The catecholamines, those homones produced from the

amino acids phenylalanine and tyrosine, appear to be particularly relevant. In his book *Life Extension*, American research scientist Durk Pearson notes how increasing the levels of noradrenalin and dopamine – two products of phenylalanine's metabolic pathway – increases sexual enthusiasm and activity. The catecholamines are also thought to regulate the release of an aphrodisiac hormone from the hypothalamus called lutenising hormone releasing hormone (LHRH). We'll examine several case histories of men and women who have successfully used these substances to energise their sex lifes in Chapter 12.

Fat Facts

Another relevant neurotransmitter is acetylcholine (ACTH). This is created from a product of fatty acid metabolism called lecithin which in turn is manufactured from the essential polyunsaturated fatty acids. These fatty acid-based chemicals are among the most widely used substances of animal metabolism. As well as acting as the precursors of lecithin, they create the immensely important short-lived regulatory hormones, the prostaglandins; form the fluid structure of the cell wall; convert external stimuli such as light into electrical nerve messages; and regulate the levels of cholesterol in the body.

These substances also help to moisten and lubricate the body's soft connective tissue and membranes including areas such as the vagina. It is this lubrication that makes the repeated penetrative action of the penis a pleasurable sensation rather than a painful, rasping one. We will see in chapter 4 how these highly reactive fatty acid chemicals are very vulnerable to damage and destruction from the free radicals. To prevent this the body calls upon an arsenal of antioxidant substances including the sulphur-based amino acids, beta carotene, vitamins C and E, and several minerals, foremost amongst them being selenium. Many of these substances are also necessary in the formation of the free-radical quenching enzymes, superoxide dismutase and glutathione peroxidase. Healthy supplies of all these nutrients, therefore, are absolutely necessary for 'well lubricated' sex organs.

Metabolic Militants

One of the reasons put forward for the thinning and drying of the vagina so characteristic of the menopause is that a genetic clock seems to signal to the body to decrease its population of the free-radical quenching enzymes. Some researchers think that the increasing vulnerability to free-radical damage that results causes much more than just thinning and drying of the vagina. Free radicals attack every part of the body's metabolism, even the genetic coding, DNA and RNA. This is probably why the older a woman becomes the greater the likelihood of giving birth to a baby suffering from a genetic disorder such as Down's syndrome; what starts off as one chance in many thousands of delivering a Down's syndrome baby in the early twenties, declines to no more than one in a hundred by the time the mother has reached 40.

In terms of understanding the full implications of the nature of free-radical activity we are still at the early stages. However, knowing the effects that it does have on sexual performance there are many nutritional measures we can take to protect ourselves from them as fully as possible, as you'll discover.

Other Nutrients

Other chemicals closely involved in vaginal lubrication are niacin (B3) and vitamin B6. B6 also works in tandem with the mineral zinc in promoting sexual health and wellbeing. Concentrated in the prostate gland, which is situated just below the bladder, zinc is a vital part of sperm production. Some nutritionists speculate that zinc may serve a similar role in the prostate gland to that of iodine in the thyroid. It is widely recognised that an iodine deficiency causes the thyroid to swell, leading to the condition known as goitre. Swollen prostate – a condition common in middle-aged men and those in later life – could be at least partly attributable to zinc deficiency. Bearing in mind that it's feasible for a man to ejaculate more zinc in his sperm than he absorbs (especially if his diet is high in processed foods, he smokes, and has sex often) the goitre parallel is a distinct possibility.

At any rate, few argue that healthy zinc levels are important for good, satisfying sex. In addition to its function in the prostate, Carl Pfeiffer, head of the Brain Bio Institute in

Princeton, has found that zinc and B6 help the sex organs to develop as well as making sexual intercourse and masturbation more physically intense, gratifying experiences.

Apart from its close ties with zinc in the prostate gland, niacin (B3) also has other relevant functions. For instance, when taken as a supplement it often causes a temporary hot flushing sensation. The recipient can turn a bright red which, in company, can be hilarious since they appear highly embarrassed. Where does the connection with sex lie? Well, not with the embarrassment. The cause of the flushing is the dilation of blood capillaries in the skin which make more blood course to the skin surface leading to the redness and increased warmth. Niacin and B6 cause this dilation thanks to a chemical interaction with an amino acid called histidine. When the three react with each other they create another substance that we've already met: histamine. Since histamine is central to orgasm, healthy levels of niacin and B6 are also required. And since almost every nutrient we've seen here is related to every other in a great metabolic merry-go-round you can see how important it is to get a good blend of nutrients rather than simply taking one and hoping for the best.

We've already covered a fair amount of ground in these first two chapters. Hopefully you now understand why nutrition is so important for a happy, healthy sex life. The remainder of the book will show how you can use these biochemical wonder workers to energise your sex life. Good sex, though, is more than simply having an erection or experiencing intensely pleasurable orgasms. To achieve these the mind and body should ideally function at a peak of mental and physical vitality. For the next three chapters, therefore, we'll see what measures you can take to scale this peak. Chapter by chapter we will build up a practical and effective nutritional programme for achieving increased mental clarity and enthusiasm, and greater energy, stamina, strength, and attractiveness.

Summary

While mental balance undoubtedly influences your level of sexual performance it is wrong to imagine that any sexual difficulties you experience are solely the result of mental or emotional problems and therefore beyond your influence. Satisfying sex also depends on a satisfactory supply of relevant nutrients and for this reason nutritional supplements can make an important difference to the quality of your sex life.

Part 2
The Vitality Foundation Course

In chapters 1 and 2, we wandered far into the microscopic highways and byeways of the body's metabolic pathways, those biochemical mazes where each meandering branch of the trail forges a new substance crucial to your health and wellbeing. We saw how these pathways are 'paved' with groups of nutrients which must be obtained from our diets: amino acids, fatty acids, vitamins, minerals, and carbohydrate. And we saw how, without these nutrients, the pathways are quickly blocked, the production of important chemicals declines, and the result is a loss of vitality. As we discovered, blockages of this kind have many causes, including the shortage of raw materials through inadequate diet and poor digestion, stress, pollution, illness, and injury. And, as well as reducing your general vitality, they quickly impair your experience and enjoyment of sex.

The remainder of this book is devoted to finding ways not just of unblocking the metabolic pathways but, if you like, of 'resurfacing' them, of making them more efficient, productive, and vibrant than anything you have ever been used to. This will, in turn, provide tremendous dividends in terms of sexual energy, stamina, performance, sensitivity, and fulfilment. From chapter 6 onwards we will look closely at enhancing those metabolic pathways closely involved with sexual functions. In the next three chapters, though, we'll look at the more general needs of your body and how to achieve both emotional and physical wellbeing. You may feel that concentrating on ways of achieving a high level of overall vitality has very little to do with a book on good sex. Alternatively you may already feel in the peak of health. If so then by all means pass straight to chapter 6.

For the rest of us, whose energy levels are not all they should be, whose resistance to infection is lower, and susceptibility to stress higher, who suffer from bout of anxiety and fatigue, periods of physical sluggishness and mental confusion, the following chapters constitute a foundation course in achieving good and longlasting health. It's this sort of wellbeing that will, in turn, provide the springboard to a fuller, more vibrant, and fulfilling sex life. And in case you don't think the two are related, look at the following example.

Selling the Sex Life Short

Dave is a sales manager in London. Typically he leaves his suburban house by 7.30 a.m., after bolting down a cup of coffee and a bowl of cereal, to drive the 40 congested, exhaust-fumed miles to work. He can be a considerate driver but rush-hour traffic intoxicates him, filling him with intolerance and impatience. The smallest incursion from a fellow driver, pulling across in front of him from an adjacent lane, perhaps, is met by the belligerent fanfare of his car horn and a lexicon of schoolboy swear-words. In this way he spends an hour and a half driving to work every day, his gorge rising inside him like a filling cistern.

Once at work he switches on his desktop coffee machine, gulps a cup down immediately, pours himself another, then, slumped over his desk, addresses himself to his monthly sales figures. Today, the figures are well short of predictions and he feels the familiar icy tautness of anxiety in his stomach. The thought of the afternoon's meeting with his managing director makes him start to perspire. The boss will want an explanation for the figures and he has only a couple of hours to find out what has gone wrong. Reviewing his figures region by region he discovers that a sales rep he was personally responsible for appointing has performed especially badly. His stomach tightens and he feels his heart start to hammer in his chest.

He works through lunch without getting anything from the canteen. The work is too important and he hasn't much of an appetite. A colleague pokes his head around the door to ask if he wants a game of squash after work. 'Too busy,' he answers, 'another time.'

The meeting in his managing director's office. He can hear his blood pounding in his temples as he reviews the figures. His head is on the block and his mind races to pre-empt his boss's questions. Partly placated, the boss asks for a revised interim sales plan by tomorrow morning. Dave spends the remainder of the day working on the new plan, pushing himself to finish the work despite increasing fatigue and an inability to concentrate. He leaves the office finally at 8.30 p.m. and trudges around the corner to a pub for a pint and a steak-and-kidney pie. Driving home, his mind reviews the same sales figures time and time again like a film caught in an endlessly repeating loop.

He is home by 10 and he and his wife, Rose, go straight to bed. Curled up under their duvet, they attempt to make love. But he feels no desire. His arms and legs feel so heavy and he is almost embarrassed by her ardour and his inability to respond. He rolls over and falls asleep. This has been the pattern for several months now. On those few occasions when they have made love, it has been mechanical and passionless and Dave has literally just gone through the motions.

Let's look at the sort of lifestyle that has led to this lack of sexual fulfilment:

- he does no exercise; on an average day he might walk a total of 200 yards, the rest of the time he sits in his car or slumps over his desk
- he lives under almost perpetual stress, whether it's driving to work or operating in the pressure-cooker of his job
- his diet is appalling; discounting cups of coffee, his food is overrefined and undernourishing.

All in all, it's no wonder their sex life is non-existent. The combination of physical confinement, intense stress, and terribly inadequate nutrition would be enough to deprive Casanova of his sexual appetite.

Dave and Rose's sex life has been marvellous in the past and could be again. However, while he abuses his mind and body the way he does this couple will continue to suffer the frustration and discontent of unfulfilling sex.

Dave's is only one example – and not a particularly extreme

one at that – of the sort of problems that will undermine the vitality necessary for good sex. Such problems affect people of all ages, of both sexes, and of most lifestyles. The chances are that they affect you. This is why merely taking those nutrients known specifically to stimulate sex is not enough.

Ensuring a good sex life means overhauling your entire way of living. That's why the next three chapters will tackle each of the three problems pinpointed in Dave's story: the stress, the bad diet, and the lack of exercise.

First, in chapter 3, we'll examine the importance of emotional wellbeing to good sex and the way that common problems such as Dave's stress interfere with it. Then we'll see what happens when you ply the emotion-related metabolic pathways with their key nutrients, helping to achieve the positive mental outlook, the enthusiasm, the energy, and the responsiveness necessary for good sex.

Chapter 3
The Most Important Sex Organ

Question: *which part of the body is the most important sex organ?*
Answer: *the brain.*

Admittedly, it's not the first part of the body you would think of. However, as we've seen, sex depends first and foremost not on physical attributes but on a subtly balanced state of emotions, wavering like a see-saw on its fulcrum between feelings such as excitement and desire on one side and relaxation and tranquillity on the other. Furthermore, sexual arousal itself starts in the brain, with fragile emotional flutters triggering the chain reaction that leads to the powerful physical responses. It's natural, therefore, that if you suffer from problems that interfere with your mental and emotional stability – such as depression and anxiety – then your sex life will be severely affected. A positive, optimistic, and balanced state of mind is crucial. In this chapter we'll look at the different ways of achieving it.

Sex on the Brain

Nearly 25 per cent of all the oxygen used in the body is consumed in the brain. As the brain weighs between 2 and 3 lb and makes up only about 2 per cent of overall body weight, this makes a phenomenal ratio. It means that at all times of the day and night the brain uses more energy than any other part of the body during its day-to-day activity (much more, say, than that used by your leg muscles when walking). With such a preponderant use of energy, its fuel needs are huge and this in turn means that it uses the lion's share of the nutrients circulating in the blood stream. It stands to reason, therefore, that any shortage of nutrients will undermine the workings of the brain. This will affect emotional wellbeing and, in turn, your degree of sexual arousal. Perhaps, but not so fast . . . Let's look at an opposing argument.

In the past, when challenged with the idea that good nutrition improves emotional and mental wellbeing, health experts have countered by citing the presence of a stringently selective biological mechanism called the blood/brain barrier. Stated simply, this is a filtering mechanism, a metabolic Berlin Wall, that separates the blood capillaries carrying the oxygen and nutrients from the brain cells they serve. The reason for this barrier is that the blood, serving in its dual role of waste disposal mechanism as well as food carrier, contains numerous waste products and toxins – such as the poisonous ammonia, a common by-product of the metabolic pathways – on their way to the kidneys to be excreted. The hyperactive cells of the brain are especially sensitive to these waste products. Any contamination leads to cellular oxidation, degradation, and cell death.

The barrier acts effectively to prevent these impurities from crossing into the brain cells. At the same time it filters through measured amounts of the essential nutrients. This barrier, therefore, is supposed to ensure that as well as protecting the brain from poisoning, it supplies all the food required to power the concentrated reactions of the brain. Even if the body is starved, the blood/brain barrier ensures that the brain will be the last thing to suffer. In practice it doesn't seem to work quite as well as this. Many nutritionists and researchers now think that if the body suffers from low levels of nutrients, for whatever reason, then this will adversely affect brain activity.

So how would you know if your brain was affected by a shortage of nutrition and what would you do about it even if it was? Answering these questions means understanding the way the brain, and its constituent nerve cells, works. Then, by seeing which nutrients are needed to supply these nerve cells and so ensure that your emotions are well balanced, we can formulate a list of the most effective supplements and foods.

Nerve Messengers

The brain is composed of about 10-15 billion nerve cells (also called neurons). Philosophers, scientists, theologians, and biochemists, not to mention bizarre combinations of the above, have argued for centuries about the nature of the brain. Some insist that it is simply a mechanism for receiving and processing messages from the body about new experiences. The processing is carried out by comparing these new messages to memories of similar previous experiences (stored biochemically in coded combinations, or circuits, of cells). Finally, having compared them, it sends out orders on how to react. This, according to the argument, makes it no more than a biochemical and electronic machine; highly complex, yes, but a machine none the less. Others agree that in purely mechanistic terms the brain is indeed an intricate machine. However, they go on to suggest that it is inhabited by a quite separate entity, a mind or spirit or soul (call it what you will) to guide it – a so-called 'ghost in the machine'. Luckily, in this book, we can forget about haunted mechanisms and look at an aspect of the brain function which everybody agrees exists: the way in which brain messages are carried from one nerve cell to the next.

From the body's sensual receiving organs – the skin, eyes, ears, tongue, and nose – messages are passed up along chains of connected neurons to the brain. Here they are interpreted and orders sent out in response to the nature of the message. Imagine you are out driving and see a red light in the road in front of you: your brain receives this message and compares it to other occasions when you've encountered a red light. This triggers recollections, stored as brain circuits, of how you responded to this stimulus in the past. In fact, this particular experience has probably happened to you so many times that the memories have become an instinct. The instinct in this case is the triggering of a set of responses which are transmitted down the motor neurons. Arms, legs, and ankle muscles are ordered to contract in a coordinated fashion so that you ease your foot onto the brake while changing into a lower gear.

From sighting the red light to the muscles receiving their orders to contract around one-thirtieth of a second has elapsed. This same order of responses occurs for every physical and most mental reactions we make, from laughing at a joke to salivating at the smell of roasting food. Admittedly, we have grossly simplified the process in our description. In fact, every reaction you make to stimuli like these is a complex mixture of many different orders from the brain; hundreds of separate muscles are made to contract and relax, networks of blood vessels to dilate or constrict, enzymes and hormones secreted, and the electromagnetic pulses of the brain waves changed in intensity.

It is the way that these messages – the stimuli to the brain and the responses from it – are carried that interests us. The receiving organs are lined with incredibly sensitive nerve cell structures rich in essential fatty acids (a classic example being the retina). When these cells are exposed to a stimulus – say light to the retina – an oxidation reaction occurs, producing in turn an electric current. A helpful comparison with the current produced by the action of light on the retina is the way the photo-sensitive cell of a photographer's light meter produces electricity, causing the gauge to flicker when held up to certain strengths of light.

Let's imagine that a young man sitting in a restaurant on his own sees, sitting two tables away, a pretty young woman. The picture of this lady is transformed into an electrical impulse, then carried along the nerve branches to his brain. However, rather than passing all the way as an electrical current, the impulse must jump a series of gaps called synapses, one between each cell. The reason for these gaps is that, with so many thousands of messages each second coursing their way towards the brain, a failsafe circuit breaker is required to prevent them all from getting mixed up. After all, in the restaurant alone, the man's senses are besieged by a mass of information: the sound of fellow diners conversing, the smell of food, his sense of hunger, the taste of wine, let alone the sight of, and his response to, the attractive woman. The synapses prevent all this from scrambling into one indecipherable buzz of biochemical static.

So how does the picture of this beautiful woman, now an electrical impulse, manage to cross these failsafe gaps? Let's watch as the message passes to the tip of the nerve cell along which it is travelling. As it reaches the furthermost point of that cell, a filament-like branch jutting out into the chasm of the synaptic gulf, the tip secretes a special chemical which makes contact with the nearest point of the next cell. Contact with this chemical then produces an identical electrical message in this second cell. This pulses to its own furthermost tip before secreting a chemical to the next cell, and so on.

These chemicals are called neurotransmitters. There are many different neurotransmitters, each one carrying a different sort of message. Some are excitory, conveying anger, euphoria, and tension, others are inhibitory, acting as forerunners of relaxation, meditation, and sleep. Others cause motor responses, making muscles contract or relax. Neurotransmitters are crucial to your mental awareness, physical responsiveness, and emotional wellbeing. As far as sex is concerned, they play particularly important roles since intercourse depends on a complex interplay of not just a few neurotransmitters but very many. As we've seen, emotionally sex is an unstable balance between excitation and relaxation: too much or too little of one state or the other is not good. Likewise with the physical nature of sex: the muscular activity involved needs strong motor neuron activity, but too much tension impedes performance as effectively as too much slackness of the muscles caused by not enough motor neuron activity. It's important, therefore, to make sure that your nerve cells are well nourished with all the nutrients needed to manufacture healthly levels of each neurotransmitter.

At the time of writing, over 40 different neurotransmitters have been discovered. They are thought to be highly sensitive to fluctuations in diet and to the effects of illness, injury, and other stresses. If your nerve cells are not supplied with the raw material nutrients they need to produce their neurotransmitters, telltale signs may include torpor, lassitude, indecisiveness, and even various stages of depression. How the young man at his table responds to the sight of the young woman therefore depends to a great extent on whether or not his neurotransmitter levels are healthy or whether in some way he is suffering from a depletion of essential raw material nutrients. One of the most common causes of such a depletion, and one to which none of us is immune, is stress. What stress is and how it depresses the levels of body nutrients is what we'll look at next.

Stressing the Point

Stress is a biochemical response that has evolved to help us live. It enables us to deal emotionally and physically with extraordinary situations, which are called stressors. It is a primal life-preserving mechanism and has three distinct stages: alarm, resistance, and exhaustion. The first stage, alarm, is the body's initial reaction to a stressor. The stressor might be the threat of physical violence from a mugger, the need suddenly to jam on your car brake as a child runs out into the street in front of you, or the angry phone call from your boss demanding the sales figures that you promised yesterday. In each of these cases, the alarm triggers your 'fight-or-flight' instinct. This clears the decks for action by changing your brain waves to a much higher pitch of activity so that your attention is more narrowly focused, more quick-witted. Your breathing becomes quicker and blood is diverted from currently non-essential areas such as the gut, face, and buttocks to the heavy muscles. Your nostrils and pupils dilate and the adrenal gland starts pumping much higher levels of adrenalin into the body.

The next stage, resistance, stabilises the body's metabolic activity at this intense pitch of arousal depending on how long the stressor lasts. That threatening mugger may after all turn out to be a pacifist vegetarian wanting directions to the nearest health-food store; the child might jump back onto the safety of the pavement. In either case the removal of the threat will leave you with nothing worse than a rapidly pounding heartbeat for a short while which will quickly return to normal. On the other hand, your boss might say that unless he has the report on his desk by the end of the day you're out of a job. In this case the resistance stage will be maintained. While you work at a fever pitch of anxiety and concentration, the body's metabolism is put under enormous strain. Protein is broken apart and consumed, salt is retained, and blood cholesterol levels increased, while important co-factor minerals such as potassium are excreted. To compensate for the rapid consumption and loss of nutrients, the body begins to draw on the circulating pool of precious raw materials. Sucked into the metabolic pathways that power the stress response, they are diverted away from the other jobs they must perform in the body.

In extreme cases this high consumption level of nutrients leads to the final stage, exhaustion. In chapter 4, we'll see how this manifests itself physically through reduced immune function and therefore less resistance to disease and illness, poor digestion, and general fatigue. For now, let's see what the emotional effects are and what can be done to stave them off.

Emotional Stress

Sustained stress can cause extreme depression or anxiety. Reading this, you may want to stop and take issue with the relevance of the statement. It's all very well, you might think, talking about the debilitating effects of extreme stress, but in what way does it relate to me? A frontline soldier in battle or an undercover narcotics agent in Colombia might be subjected to sustained stress. The drain on their nutrient resources from operating constantly in a life-and-death situation could easily lead to the exhaustion stage. But in all probability, the most stressful situation that our young restaurant patron will have endured will have been the minor, everyday nightmares of clambering onto the underground or subway on a wet mid-winter morning or going to the dentist to have root-canal surgery. How could these possibly influence his approach to the young woman?

In fact, in almost everything he does he is under stress and this must affect him. In many ways it is a positive force, stimulating us all to respond more efficiently in any given situation. After all, making love is itself a stressor. But stress can also be incredibly pernicious. Try listing all those occasions during the day when something or someone has annoyed you. Think of the arguments, suppressed anger, and resentment towards boorish workmates, pedestrians who barge into you in the street, indifferent shop assistants, and sanctimonious politicians sermonising on television. List your responses to the news of the latest bomb outrage, the latest rise in mortgage interest rates, the rocketing gas and electricity bills, the screaming children. Going outside in freezing cold, wet weather is a stressor. So are cigarette smoke and excessive alcohol, calorie restriction diets, illness and injury, separation, childbirth, and bereavement. Each of these, and untold thousands more, are stressors. Each, in their small way, demand a stress response: alarm and resistance, alarm and resistance, alarm and resistance. Each, therefore, is depleting your body of its supply of nutrients. Day after day, month after month, the cumulative effect of these stressors may be every bit as sapping as the threat of a mujahadin onslaught or shadow of a drug baron.

Furthermore, as one of the actions of the stress response is to divert blood away from assisting with digestion, the more stress you undergo, the poorer your digestion will be. This means that fewer raw material nutrients will be made available for distribution through the body. So what are the results? The two most common emotional consequences are depression and anxiety. We'll look at both.

Depression

There are two basic forms of depression and both can be traced to the exhaustion stage of stress. The first, reactive depression, is, as its name suggests, a direct response to a particular stressor. It may be a bereavement, the loss of a job, involvement in a major accident or disaster. Whatever it is, it causes such a powerful trauma that the nutrient reserves are quickly depleted. Reactive depression is a common result of shock. The second form is called endogenous depression and it defies being liked to any specific causes. However, many health experts look upon it as a consequence of the barrage of ministressors that we must each weather every day. Some people have fewer resources with which to withstand the nutritional depletions these stressors cause than others.

What each of these forms of depression has in common is that they lead to a number of stereotyped symptoms that include torpor, fatigue, an inability to act positively, self-hatred, and a craving for solitude. A well-known comedian calls these responses 'the cold-bath syndrome': lying in the tub, you feel the water gradually go tepid as it laps around your skin in little chilly flutters; it makes you feel increasingly miserable and, because of that, you can't rouse yourself to climb out; instead, as it gets colder, you become even more miserable, making it even more difficult to escape. This little scene that we've all experienced illustrates perfectly the self-perpetuating nature of depression, the way that everything seems to lack meaning, the way any action, no matter how great or small, seems pointless. Most of us snap ourselves out of these situations. However, the more our metabolic pathways are drained by continual stress, the harder it gets to fight these feelings.

Not surprisingly, in these cases, the idea of having sex is not only unappealing but impossible. A case in point is the story of Louise, a maths teacher in an inner-city high school.

Staff shortages and lack of resources put teachers under severe emotional strain. Like her colleagues, Louise is expected to deal with ever-growing classes of mostly recalcitrant children. Often, rather than bring in supply teachers to cover for those absent through ill health (and this number increases weekly), the school tries to economise by getting the staff to cover by sacrificing their 'free' periods. For Louise, this means that she has even less time to prepare for lessons and recover from other stressful and tiring encounters with her children. The atmosphere, she says, is one of low morale, declining self-esteem, and great stress.

Over a period of roughly four months, Louise felt herself sinking into what she ironically describes as 'the slough of despond'. 'I would go in and some days be so miserable that I was totally absorbed and obsessed with my own little world of woe,' she says. 'I just didn't care. I got tired easily and very tearful. Everything looked bleak, there didn't seem to be a way out.' Not surprisingly, Louise's relationship with her boyfriend, Robin, suffered. 'I couldn't communicate what I was feeling. I hated him touching me and couldn't understand why he should possibly want to have sex with me. It just meant nothing. I just wanted to sleep when I got home. Not talk, or eat, or make love, just sleep.'

She did, however, read in a women's magazine in the staff room about the antidepressant effects of a particular nutritional supplement. On impulse she went into a health-food shop and bought a cannister of the product. The supplement in question is one we met briefly in chapter 1: the essential amino acid called phenylalanine. 'I took it twice a day,' she says, 'and, honestly, the change in me was so sudden. I felt galvanised. I had so much more energy. I was alert, I felt refreshed, I had stamina. I felt the way you do when you wake up in a sun-filled room after a deep, refreshing sleep.'

Phenylalanine affected Louise so dramatically because it supplements precisely those neurotransmitters which are depleted by stress. Here's how.

Phenylalanine is the parent molecule – that is, it sits at the start of a metabolic pathway – of a group of substances called catecholamines. These chemicals are known to be severely depleted by stress and their loss was one of the first physical causes of depression that scientists successfully pinpointed. The most important chemicals in the catecholamine group are the hormones noradrenalin and adrenalin. Because these two chemicals are secreted at high levels by the stress response, the raw materials necessary for producing them (phenylalanine and the other co-factor nutrients) are used up much more quickly than normal. Yet, paradoxically, it is when you suffer from sustained stress that your levels of noradrenalin and adrenalin need to be at their healthiest to help you resist it. Both are vital for helping to stimulate mental clarity and emotional wellbeing. Whether you laugh at a joke, run for a bus, or argue, you need noradrenalin and adrenalin to arouse your response. Not surprisingly, they are crucial in assisting sexual arousal.

There are, in fact, two forms of phenylalanine: 'D' and 'L'. The two are molecular mirror images of each other. It is usually the 'L' form of amino acids which affect our biochemistry. However, in phenylalanine's case, while the 'L' stimulates production of the catecholamines, the 'D' form has a different but key effect: it enhances the effects of a group of naturally occurring morphine-like substances called endorphins. Endorphins are produced at the same time as adrenalin. They are the chemicals responsible for the euphoria experienced by athletes as they pass through the pain barrier. Usually, though, endorphins are rapidly broken down by enzymes so that such effects are short-lived. D-phenylalanine, however, actually blocks the action of these destructive enzymes, in turn prolonging the effects of the endorphins.

The result is an automatic release of tension, calmer, smoother brain-wave patterns and a generally powerful and positive antidepressant effect. Phenylalanine is often sold in a form that combines both D and L called DL-phenylalanine, or DLPA for short. Among the enormous advantages of taking DLPA over conventional antidepressants is that it naturally strengthens the metabolic pathways. Antidepressants, while stimulating catecholamine neurotransmitter production, then prevent their reabsorption after use by the nerve endings. This in turn leads to a progressive depletion of the raw material nutrients needed to create noradrenalin and adrenalin. Consequently, the victim has to continue taking antidepressants, setting in motion the cycle of dependency.

Extensive double-blind tests (where neither patient nor researcher know who is receiving which substance) have proved DLPA to be at least as effective at relieving depression as imipramine, one of the most popular antidepressant drugs.

In chapter 1 we wrote about the importance of co-factors in the metabolic pathways. Substrate chemicals don't miraculously metamorphose into other chemicals on their own. The changes are due to the interaction of co-factor vitamins and minerals. Therefore, when strengthening any pathway through supplementation, such as with DLPA, it is wise to complement it with supplements of the relevant co-factors. In the case of DLPA the co-factors are magnesium and copper, together with vitamins B1, B3, B6, folic acid, and C. From time to time throughout the book we'll present you with a list of nutrients that we suggest you follow for achieving a particular response. Since we're brought up to think of medicines in terms of one-pill palliatives, a list of five or more separate supplements might put you off. Try not to let it, though. And if you need any incentive just look what it did for Louise: 'Yes, work is a lot better; at least I find I'm able to cope, which has to be seen as a victory. But better by far is that things have improved terrifically between me and Robin. After a really bad time of it, our physical relationship is wonderful and to be honest I think I'm tiring him out a bit.'

Stress without the Stressor

While stemming from the same stereotypical stress response, anxiety is almost the opposite of depression. Whereas depression can be caused by the exhaustion of those nutrients necessary for maintaining the stress response – the catecholamines – anxiety occurs when the body secretes the catecholamines in response to a non-existent stressor. With the secretion of adrenalin your heartbeat increases, you perspire, your scalp tightens and hairs rise up on your skin, blood is moved away from the stomach to fuel and nourish the larger muscles – causing the characteristic queasy switchback sensation as well as lowering the rate of digestion – and your brain waves change from tranquil alpha-wave activity to excited beta wave. So if there is nothing to respond to, what causes this?

The best way to answer that question is to look at an anxiety-causing situation. Late one evening a woman is on her way home after working overtime stock-taking at the supermarket. Her path takes her through an unlit pedestrian subway where she is accosted by a drunkard, beaten, and robbed. After a night in hospital she returns with the police to the scene of the crime. However, despite being in the presence of friends, despite the fact that it is now a sunny morning, the trauma has been so great that her stress response fires in preparation for an identical attack. Obviously none will happen, but she is now conditioned to experience the worst: her heartbeat races, her breathing comes in short gasps, and she is almost sick from the tension in her stomach.

This is an anxiety response. And although it is often triggered by fear of a specific situation – be it this mugging, or incessant pressure at work from your boss, involvement in a motor accident, or being made unemployed – it often invades every aspect of your waking life.

A close friend of ours, Alec, who works in a firm of chartered accountants as a junior executive, recently found himself the victim of extreme anxiety. Soon after joining his firm he was presented with a *fait accompli*: all three senior colleagues in his section defected to a competitor. He was effectively left to run the section with his very limited experience until replacements could be appointed. 'It was very, very frightening,' he remembers. 'I made a hash of everything. I had clients phoning up for advice on topics I knew nothing about, others demanding meetings to review complicated consultancy problems, senior partners breathing down my neck wanting to know why I wasn't doing one thing or another. I felt I was drowning.'

The first inkling he had of problems was that queasy sense of dread clenched in his stomach. 'Then it seemed to work its way up. A few days after this my heart began to pound, then a little later I started suffering from insomnia – not just unable to get off right away, but no sleep at all for several nights at a go. Every phone call in my office was a cause of dread. After a while I just sat at my desk taking my pulse all day. I was paralysed with anxiety and obsessed with its effects.'

Happiness is an Amino Acid

Happily, relief lay in the form of a nutritional supplement of the amino acid tryptophan. Like phenylalanine, tryptophan is a precursor of one of the major neurotransmitters. Unlike the excitory adrenalin, tryptophan produces an inhibitory neurotransmitter called serotonin. Serotonin is one of the body's natural tranquillisers and is secreted prior to dropping off to sleep. Although tryptophan supplements help to overcome insomnia – for which Alec was supremely grateful – their effects are much more far-reaching. Anxiety sufferers are typically low in serotonin and when tryptophan supplements are administered many of their symptoms, such as the racing heartbeat and queasy stomach, are alleviated. Tryptophan also encourages the production of alpha brain waves to counteract the racing, obsessive nature of the beta waves which are one of the major causes of insomnia.

At this point, however, our story takes on a sour note. At the time of writing, tryptophan has been withdrawn from sale on both sides of the Atlantic in any nutritional supplement of which it is the major constituent. This is the explanation. Free form amino acids are produced in two grades: pharmaceutical (which are pure enough to be given intravenously) and food (which are produced mainly as animal supplementation). In mid-1988 a certain Japanese company produced a contaminated batch of food-grade tryptophan which found its way into oral supplements taken by people. It caused fatigue and high levels of a particular type of white blood cell called eisoniphil.

Although limited to one company's production, this amino acid, which is essential for life and has been used safely for decades by millions of people, received a bout of horrendous publicity and was withdrawn from sale. Dark rumours have circulated of pressure brought to bear on the FDA to sanction the withdrawal by pharmaceutical companies that manufacture serotonin derivatives and are anxious to muscle in on tryptophan's territory. At this stage it is impossible to predict the eventual outcome and say whether tryptophan will be reinstated or not. None the less, we believe that oral supplements of tryptophan made from the pharmaceutical-grade quality, as most are, carry no risk of contamination. For this reason, we will refer to tryptophan on occasion throughout this book. Even though it is not currently available we can only hope that by the time the book is published it will be.

> For proof of tryptophan's efficacy we only have to look at its effects on Alec's anxiety condition. He took it over a couple of weeks, and his acute anxiety gradually faded. 'There were times when I felt the pressure mounting up – my heart racing, my stomach telling me I'd just gone over the top of the world's biggest roller coaster. Then I'd take a capsule of tryptophan and feel much calmer, although not drowsy either; just relaxed.'

It's worth mentioning here that tryptophan, like all the supplements mentioned in the book, is not a medicine. It is simply a natural food with natural effects helping to strengthen the metabolic pathways. Natural sources include spirulina, dried seaweed, parmesan cheese and sesame seeds.

Phenylalanine and tryptophan are probably the most effective supplements you can take to help you overcome any problems of stress or anxiety. However, there are a number of other supplements that many people also find useful in promoting mental and emotional stability. Very briefly we'll look at each of these three in turn.

Dust Cart and Brain Fuel

Probably the most effective of this subsidiary group is the amino acid glutamine. It has been found to increase mental clarity, alertness, and concentration by acting jointly as a detoxifier and fuel source. You must remember that the brain is a phenomenal power-house of metabolic activity. This means that in addition to the messages shooting back and forth around the neural networks there is a great deal of waste material. Much of this waste material takes the form of ammonia, which is a mixture of nitrogen and hydrogen atoms and a by-product of the breakdown of spent amino acids, as well well as being a metabolic poison. A build-up of ammonia – perhaps due to stress or anxiety, or even long work hours – interferes with concentration, causes exaggerated mood swings, irritability, confusion, and poor memory.

This ammonia is disposed of by a metabolic pathway called

the urea cycle, which converts the toxin to urea then excretes it harmlessly in the urine. The key component of this reaction in the brain is glutamic acid, an offshoot of glutamine. If, for whatever reason, there is not enough glutamic acid to convert the ammonia then behavioural problems will result. The causes of this shortfall might be dietary or they might be due to excessive brain activity producing more ammonia than the urea cycle can cope with. Jet lag is a common cause of such problems since it disrupts the brain's normal sleep patterns. And, as nutritionist Richard Passwater says, 'the shortage of glutamine in the diet or glutamic acid in the brain results in brain damage due to excess ammonia or a brain that can never get into gear.'

Glutamine also doubles as a brain fuel, supplying a source of energy similar to that of glucose. A glutamine supplement, therefore, is well worth considering if you feel befuddled, if it takes numerous cups of coffee to start you off in the morning and if you have difficulty sustaining your concentration levels and interest in your work or your relationships. Try 200mg with each meal together with vitamins B6, C, and folic acid to encourage the conversion in the brain to glutamic acid.

G-Force

Two other amino acids, both also starting with the letter 'g', are the last supplements we'll meet in this chapter. One, glycine, is the most common of the 22 amino acids in the body. It is used in the spinal cord as a neuro-inhibitor, calming jerky, uncoordinated movement. People find it especially useful if they feel nervous and clumsy in company particularly with a person of the opposite sex. The same is true of gamma-amino-butyric acid, or GABA for short, which is often used to soothe manic behaviour and acute agitation. Start with around 250mg a day together with the important vitamin co-factors: B3, C, and folic acid.

Tying up the Ends

So how does all this information relate to you? You probably don't suffer from depression or anxiety. You are probably well balanced, fairly optimistic, sometimes up, sometimes down. However, the point about these supplements is not that they can help you if these emotional problems occur (although they obviously can), but that they can help to inject an even greater zest, enthusiasm, and a satisfying emotional roundness into your life than you might already enjoy. Don't think of them merely as solutions for anxiety and depression. If they have such an effect on those problems, then think how they can potentiate your own attitude towards your life in general and your love life in particular.

Although phenylalanine and tryptophan stimulate starkly different neurotransmitter responses, they do not oppose each other, but complement each other perfectly. Phenylalanine helps to arouse you emotionally and physically, tryptophan tempers that arousal, making the experience richer and mellower, both more receptive and sensitive. Add glutamine, glycine, and GABA to this list and you have a world-beating formula for emotional wellbeing.

As for our young, besotted diner, there's no doubting that his brain chemical levels are healthy and well supplied. He relishes the challenges and thrills of the unknown, particularly new relationships. Admiring from afar the poise and self-possession of the female patron, his mind's eye watches their relationship develop in a series of tableaux. He pictures passionate lovemaking, long walks on deserted beaches in the coppery sunset, travelling together in foreign countries, and even a candlelit dinner in this very restaurant to celebrate the anniversary of their first meeting. He steels himself to cross the floor to introduce himself, his mind clear and alert, the fear and anxiety of a rebuff under control. Unfortunately, no amount of good nutrition prevents the woman's husband from emerging from the men's room at that moment and seating himself next to her. Never mind; if only thwarted ambition was the only thing that stood in the way of good sex.

Summary

Good sex needs a foundation of emotional wellbeing, as free as possible from stress symptoms such as anxiety and depression. You can help to ensure this level of wellbeing by using a cross section of those nutrients that enable the metabolic pathways to manufacture the relevant stress-beating neurotransmitters.

These nutrients are:

1 **Phenylalanine** For stimulating the excitory brain chemicals noradrenalin and adrenalin; or DLPA which, in addition to stimulating these chemicals, will also help to simulate the painkilling and euphoria-inducing endorphins. Either of these forms of amino acid act as powerful antidepressants and should be taken with the co-factors magnesium, copper, B1, B3, B6, C, and folic acid.
2 **Tryptophan** By stimulating the inhibitory and sleep-inducing neurotransmitter, serotonin, this acts as protection against anxiety.
3 **Glutamine** By detoxifying waste ammonia and acting as a brain fuel it aids clearer, sharper thought.
4 **Glycine and GABA** Both of these soothe agitated behaviour.

2, 3 or 4 should be taken with the co-factors B6, C, and folic acid.

Chapter 4
The Body in Question

Now that we've seen some effective nutritional measures you can take to help achieve the degree of emotional balance crucial for an enthusiastic approach to sex, let's see what we can do to charge up the body in the same way. Physical vitality – a state in which the body's glands and organs work at peak efficiency, in which toxins are eliminated quickly and efficiently, and in which a ready supply of raw material nutrients are on hand to power the metabolic pathways – is essential to being able to perform sexually. However, day in, day out the body has to fight off attacks from numerous factors that work to undermine this state of vitality, chipping away at it like saboteurs a tiny little bit at a time. Seemingly innocuous, their effects are insidious and cumulative. Over a period of time they can sap your energy, reduce your immune response, cause widespread imbalances within the metabolic pathways, trigger degenerative diseases, and deplete your body of many of the raw materials necessary for ensuring sexual vitality. To guard against them you have to be vigilant.

In this chapter, therefore, we'll look briefly at some of the commonest such threats to health. Then we'll suggest certain supplements for protecting and energising your metabolic pathways. These are the raw materials necessary for increasing your resistance to these unseen enemies and for providing extra energy with which to tackle the demands of your life. As with the techniques we looked at for achieving emotional stability, they can have far-reaching and positive effects on your sex life.

If, having read this chapter, you feel you want to discover more about particular problems, and the way in which a careful choice of supplements can help you, refer to the book list on page 169.

Gut to Get You into My Life

The stomach and intestines are of enormous importance for your overall health. Every raw material needed for the metabolic pathways, except for oxygen, is supplied by the digestive process. In the stomach, powerful hydrochloric acid starts dismantling the food as well as activating a digestive enzyme called pepsin. On average, 15 per cent of protein digestion is carried out here before the food is passed on to the duodenum and small intestine. There, other powerful digestive enzymes are secreted from the pancreas to complete the process. Once stripped away from the food, the individual molecules are then absorbed through the intestinal mucosa, or gut lining, and passed into the blood stream.

The quality of the raw materials reaching the metabolic pathways, then, depends not only on the quality of the food you consume – how fresh it is, how varied, how unrefined, how rich in essential nutrients – but also on the efficiency of your digestion. Therefore, a healthily functioning gut, one in which all the necessary digestive acids and enzymes are present, where the passage of food is rapid, and where the gut lining is in good condition, is crucial to the body's overall vitality. It determines how quickly your tissue will be able to grow and rejuvenate, your emotional wellbeing, and physical vigour. Alternatively, poor digestion leads to a variety of problems. It causes sluggishness, fatigue, and emotional instability. It can cause bad breath, skin complaints such as eczema, migraine, and increased susceptibility to illness and disease. Worryingly, many things can interfere with your digestion, one or more of which might be affecting you right now. Let's see what they are.

One of the most common contributing causes of poor digestion is cigarette smoke. It's widely known that smoking destroys lung tissue (leading to bronchitis, emphysema, and lung cancer), oxidises vitamins, increases the heavy metal content in the blood, and raises cholesterol levels. What is less well known is that cigarette smoke also depresses the body's levels of stomach acid. It's unclear how heavy the smoking needs to be but, bearing in mind the effect that even passive smoking has in promoting lung diseases, it might not need to be very great. Other causes of stomach acid loss include sustained stress and anxiety, problems which, as we've already seen, are very common. And since stomach acid activates pepsin, with the loss of the acid the pepsin levels will likewise drop.

Since these two substances alone are responsible for the lion's share of protein digestion, their decline means that far greater amounts of undigested food will pass onto the duodenum. This in turn will leave the intestinal enzymes much larger amounts of food to digest than they are capable of. It is the equivalent of telling a demolition crew not to use their wrecking ball to knock a building down but instead to use their mallets for the task. Just as the demolition crew will exhaust themselves with very little to show for the exertion, so the intestinal enzymes will become depleted in trying to digest so much food.

The results of this will be fourfold:

- First, much of the important raw materials required by the body from the food will not be released into the blood.
- Second, instead of being digested this food will start to putrefy, causing the release of harmful toxins. Some of these toxins, such as the nitrosamines, are potentially carcinogenic, while others such as octopamine displace certain neurotransmitters in the nerve cells causing alarming emotional swings.
- Third, the pancreas will attempt to secrete more digestive enzymes to cope with the extra undigested food, diverting amino acids and co-factors from other important tasks in the body. This diversion may have ramifications throughout the metabolic pathways: it may mean that repair and regeneration of tissue declines, causing symptoms such as split nails and dry, flaky skin, muscles that tire easily and take longer to recover after exercise, and cuts and bruises that take longer to heal. It may also mean that toxic waste products, such as ammonia, are not removed as quickly as they should be, causing joint stiffness and the appearance of small pustules on the skin.
- Fourth and last, the loss of digestive enzymes will allow a colony of potentially troublesome immigrants living in an uneasy truce with the gut to rebel.

These immigrants are the intestinal bacteria, living organisms in their own right which the body uses to help digest its food. Usually they are important allies. They create a barrier between the gut wall and other dangerous micro-organisms present in some tap water and poorly prepared food. They also produce some complex B vitamins, help the assimilation of minerals, and allow for a quicker passage of waste products. However, without the constraining effects of the enzymes, certain virulent strains of these bacteria will start to flourish out of control. This will itself lead to further putrefaction of the food.

Furthermore, any yeast – traces of which can be found in all foods – will also make the carbohydrate in your food start to ferment. Cases have been recorded where victims of excessive intestinal flora have actually become drunk from eating carbohydrate foods such as bread or potatoes. Even in less extreme cases such a problem can cause behavioural difficulties, fatigue, irritability, anxiety, and stress. It will also create a continual craving for carbohydrate foods particularly of the refined variety. And, of course, it will also increase your need for a drink. This problem can become a self-perpetuating cycle: the more carbohydrate you eat the greater your craving for carbohydrate becomes.

To sum up, then, poor digestion can result from a variety of all-too-common causes. Smoke, drink, refined food, and stress can all contribute. And once it takes hold it can cripple your general sense of wellbeing. As well as the mood changes caused by the release of toxins into the blood stream, other symptoms to look out for include a reduced resistance to infection, a continuing sense of bloatedness and overweight, bad skin (eczema and psoriasis are common symptoms of digestive difficulties), flatulence, body odour, and fetid stools. You will also feel heavier, less fit, and more easily fatigued. It doesn't take much imagination to realise the effect these problems will have on your sex life.

Happily there are several steps you can take to improve the health and efficiency of your digestive system. One of the most effective is to use an amino acid supplement complex. Now widely available in health-food shops, this is a blend of about 20 amino acids used by the body to create its entire range of protein structures, from muscle and enzymes to DNA and antibodies. Since all the digestive enzymes are themselves proteins manufactured from amino acids, the complex helps replace the materials lost by poor digestion and those drained by the efforts of the pancreas to compensate. Furthermore, as individual 'raw materials' themselves, the amino acids in this complex are absorbed straight through the gut lining without having to call upon the protein-digesting enzymes to digest them.

It is also important, of course, that the food you eat is of the richest and most natural quality. Try to reduce your intake of refined foods systematically. Devise a plan in which the amount of bread, cakes, pasta, biscuits, and sweets are slowly cut, while substituting what remains with wholemeal alternatives. Eat more foods that contain complex fibre to help speed the passage of digested materials through the gut and so safeguard yourself against food putrefaction. Bran might not be the best choice of fibre if you suffer from poor digestion because, although it can absorb much of the moisture in the bowel, it can combine with minerals, making them unavailable. Its roughness can also cause the gut to secrete mucus in order to protect itself. Rather than bran, eat lots of fresh fruits and vegetables as well as pulses such as lentils. If you can find a regular supply of organic fruit and vegetables, so much the better. The passage of the food through your gut will also be helped by eating foods high in essential fatty acids, such as trout, salmon, flax oil, and sunflower seeds. Their oils literally lubricate the gut lining.

However, no matter how well they eat, most people's guts retain certain residues of poisonous waste products. Such waste usually accumulates over many years, continuing to putrefy and undermine the body's overall vitality. In order to eliminate these potentially damaging chemicals, people are turning increasingly to the benefits of colonic irrigation. In essence this is a cleansing of the bowel with a stream of warm water by means of a pipe that is placed in the sphincter. It sounds awful and the experience can, admittedly, be unpleasant. The amount of crusty, tarlike waste that is usually removed, though, can be astonishing. Because the procedure removes everything in the colon, many therapists give healthy intestinal bacteria to the patient afterwards. Colonic irrigation is carried out by therapists and probably the best place to find out if there is one near you is through your health practitioner or local health-food shop.

Separating Fat from Fiction

Recommending that you increase your intake of fatty acids – the building blocks of fats and oils – as we did in the paragraph before last might seem a little odd in a chapter on how to improve your overall health. After all, we know that fat is bad for us. It causes obesity and heart disease, clogging up the arteries like last autumn's leaves in the guttering. In fact, an intake of certain specific fatty acids is every bit as important as consuming good-quality protein. Fatty acids have a tendency to disperse in water to form a fine film little more than a molecule thick (look at the way a droplet of oil spreads out to form a thin iridescent layer on the water's surface). This, and their insolubility, means that they make up the bulk of cellular membranes, the walls which permit certain nutrients to cross while restricting others.

Of course, we're not talking about any old fat. We're talking in fact about certain specific varieties with low melting points and a degree of chemical reactivity that is almost magical. It is this variety of fatty acid which ensures the fluidity and flexibility of the cell membrane, allowing the important nutrients to cross into the cell. It is also these cells that trigger and regulate many of the most important chemical reactions of the living process. These fats are known as polyunsaturated fatty acids. Simply, 'polyunsaturate' means that a fatty acid molecule has two or more vacant sites on its central carbon atom spine. The more sites it has, the more unsaturated it becomes and the more chemically reactive.

Good sources of polyunsaturated fatty acids include safflower and sunflower oils, evening primrose and borage oils, and marine oils from fatty fish. However, flax oil, the unadulterated, unrefined version of linseed oil, is the best of the lot. At the other end of the metabolic spectrum to these oils come those fatty acids found in red meats, the saturates. These have a high melting point and low level of chemical reactivity. Consumed in excess, they have a tendency to clog up the arteries by agglomerating in plaques along vessel walls, their high melting point making them solid at body temperature.

As well as maintaining the fluidity of the cell membranes, the polyunsaturates have numerous other biochemical functions. As the precursors of a group of chemicals called prostaglandins, they regulate the body on a moment-to-moment basis; they create carrier molecules called high-density lipoproteins to shuttle the saturates and cholesterol away from tissue which may be susceptible to fat agglomeration such as artery walls; they keep the circulatory system flowing freely; they act as important neurotransmitters; in short they behave in total contravention of the conventional picture we have of fat in the body. With so many ready sources of these poly-unsaturates in the shops, you would imagine that all you could possibly need was obtained from your diet.

The problem is that the chemical reactivity of these fatty acids make them highly vulnerable to attack and degradation from ordinary environmental factors such as light, heat, and oxygen. The reason a fish will rapidly go rancid, or why cod liver oil tastes revoltingly of rubber, is that the fatty acids they contain react with unseemly speed in the air to oxidise, become rancid, and create harmful toxins (in contrast, a piece of red meat will take many times longer to degrade because the saturated fatty acids it contains are so inert).

This means two things: first, much of the polyunsaturated oil we consume, such as sunflower oil, has already degraded to some extent simply from sitting in the bottle. Second, in order to extract the oil, the seeds are passed through industrial screw-presses causing intense heat and pressure, with the result that the molecular structure barely resembles its natural equivalent. And frying with these oils only increases the speed of degradation, making them virtually unusable by the body.

These sources of degraded polyunsaturates are not only found in the oils we cook with. Take a look at sunflower margarines, proudly proclaimed by their manufacturers to be high in these essential fatty acids. What the manufacturers don't tell you is that the process used to make the polyunsatu-rates solid and waxy – known as hydrogenation – actually forces some of the polyunsaturates into unnatural, and potentially toxic, configurations. A shortfall of these essential polyunsaturates has been linked to high cholesterol levels, cardiovascular illnesses, pre-menstrual tension, illnesses of the connective tissue such as rheumatism, and even, in certain pioneering studies, to cancer. Yet, if the goodness these fatty acids contain is to be protected, the oil must be kept in an opaque, airtight container in the fridge – and how many households do that?

Consequently, increasing numbers of people are now taking

supplements rich with these essential polyunsaturated fatty acids. Two varieties have emerged as especially important for your health and vitality. One is a supplement high in a fatty acid called gamma linolenic acid. This fatty acid is the precursor of the important series 1 prostaglandin, a substance that regulates water balance, hormone secretion, and blood cholesterol levels. Gamma linolenic acid has also been found to help relieve the symptoms of pre-menstrual tension, rheumatism, and joint pains, and is even recommended by some nutritionists to sufferers of multiple sclerosis. The most widely used source of this fatty acid is evening primrose oil.

A second group of important fatty acids are two called, respectively, eicosopentanoic acid and docosahexanoic acid, which are especially prevalent in marine animals. These are even more reactive than gamma linoleic acid and are especially important for the nerve endings.

These polyunsaturates also make up more complex substances called phosphatides, rather in the way that amino acids make up proteins. Some phosphatides such as lecithin and choline can also be obtained in supplement form. Furthermore, these two are precursors of a quite vital neurotransmitter called acetylcholine, a substance which plays a critical role in balancing the body between excitation and relaxation (and is, therefore, an important element in the sex response).

Let's assume that you are aware of the dangers of obtaining your sources of essential polyunsaturates from the refined oils and margarines available. You decide to cut down your fat intake as far as possible. Instead, for their therapeutic value, you take supplements of evening primrose oil and marine oil as well as eating fresh fish. Considering the remarkable nutritive qualities of the fatty acids, this should have many advantages: it may promote smoother, suppler skin, increase the freedom of movement and flexibility of your joints and connective tendons, help you think more clearly and calmly, and improve your circulation. Nutritionists believe that all this and more will be assisted by essential fatty acids.

There is a fly in the ointment, though. Because even if you follow this dietary regime religiously the fatty acids you consume will still be vulnerable to many of the ordinary day-to-day factors that have already rendered the cooking oil partially worthless. Even in the body the fatty acids are still at risk: at risk from the heavy metals carried in cigarette smoke, from alcohol and refined food, from environmental pollution such as poor-quality drinking water and high levels of carbon dioxide, from the positive ions generated by VDU screens, and from viral and bacterial infections. Even the power source of all metabolic activity, oxygen, will degrade those fatty acids.

What each of these have in common, and the reason they damage the polyunsaturates, is that they all generate biochemically ravenous and potentially toxic substances called free radicals.

Free radicals are promiscuously reactive molecules which in certain forms are crucial to the normal oxidative processes of life (that is, generating energy and causing electrical transmissions). In essence, a free radical is short of one electron, leaving it with an 'unpaired electron'. The sole aim of this solitary electron is to find a mate to balance its electronic charge and it achieves this by tearing an electron free from an adjoining molecule. This molecule is then left with an unpaired electron and tears one free from another, and so on. Forty thousand or more reactions like this can occur and, in the process, tissue is broken apart. Free radical activity has been implicated in the host of degenerative diseases and is even thought to be the cause of ageing. And, since the essential polyunsaturates are by far the most sensitive chemicals in the body, they are most at risk from this damage. Unchecked, the fatty acids will do to your body what light and oxygen do to the fish sitting on the work-top – make it go rancid.

Free radicals were recently drawn to the public's attention by a report discussing their effects on polyunsaturates. Unfortunately the report was misinterpreted as refuting the beneficial effects of polyunsaturates. What this report actually said was that polyunsaturates, due to their immense chemical sensitivity, attract free radicals like honey attracts bees. Therefore, increasing polyunsaturate levels – be it through supplementation or through eating nutritious natural sources such as fish – was likely to increase the activity of free radicals and in turn increase the likelihood of a host of degenerative diseases: cancer was mentioned. This was simplified by a tabloid paper to say that it was the polyunsaturates themselves that were to blame for these diseases.

The truth is that polyunsaturates merely happened to be in

the wrong place at the wrong time. Free radicals are the real enemies. The implication of this report, therefore, is that far from reducing your intake of polyunsaturates, you should supplement it with nutrients that will block, or quench, the effects of the free radicals. The body has evolved mechanisms to do just that, notably using enzymes called superoxide dismutase and glutathione peroxidase. However, with the explosion in environmental toxicity during this century, there is every suggestion that the body simply can't cope on its own.

The enzymes that counteract free radicals are made up of certain prominent nutrients: so-called antioxidants. These are vitamins A, C, and E, the amino acid glutathione (a mixture of the aminos cysteine, glycine, and glutamic acid), and selenium. Among the highest natural sources of selenium are onion, garlic, flour, and bread. As work at a Scottish agricultural college shows, British bakers prefer to use flour which has much lower levels of selenium in it. In the past 15 years, our average daily intake has dropped from 60 mcg to little over 40, well below the recommended daily allowances (RDAs) of many countries, although not Britain since none has been established. This is one more argument in favour of supplementation.

The supplements included in this chapter won't suddenly cause a river of vitality, strength, and athleticism to flood through you. What they will do, though, is protect you from some of the most prevalent, yet unacknowledged threats to our health today. We are all affected by factors such as environmental toxicity. Whether we like it or not they can undermine our health and interfere with our experience and enjoyment of life. These nutrients therefore make a marvellously worthwhile insurance policy. Most importantly, though, by increasing your body's vitality, they can help to make your sex life just that much more special.

Summary

Overall physical vitality is as important for good sex as mental wellbeing. Thorough, efficient digestion is a key to your body's health since it determines how well the raw materials from your food reach the metabolic pathways. A good way of achieving and maintaining digestion is by following these guidelines:

1 The complete amino acid blend; this supplies the raw materials of all the digestive enzymes.
2 A diet high in fresh fruit and vegetables, pulses, and fish, and low in processed food and red meats.
3 Supplements of polyunsaturated fatty acids such as gamma linolenic acid, flax oil, or marine oils. They must, however, be protected from the oxidising effects of free radicals by means of supplements of antioxidants such as vitamins A, E, and C, and selenium.

Chapter 5
Diving into the Water Works

We've looked at foods for the mind and foods for the body. This last chapter of our foundation course in vitality has less to do with the energising effects of food and more to do with how your body gets rid of the waste products of metabolic activity once that food has been used up. Waste elimination is essential to good health and in this chapter we'll explain just how much more vibrant and active you can feel when everything is working well.

There are a number of waste-disposal routes used by the body. These include:

- the bowels, which carry undigested nitrogenous waste products as well as other impurities returning from their trips around the circulatory system
- the kidneys and urinary tract, which filter waste products and toxins such as ammonia out of the blood and excrete them in the urine
- the lungs, which expel carbon dioxide as the by-product of energy release
- the skin – the body's largest organ – which, as we saw earlier, is a route used to extrete toxins.

We are not going to look at any of these. Rather we are going to look at the lymphatic system. This is to the body what a Georgian bay window would be to a post-modern skyscraper: namely, a relic of an earlier age fitting rather uncomfortably into something altogether more sophisticated and efficient. A relic it may be, but it can have a tremendous bearing on your health and sex life. An efficient lymphatic system ensures alertness, increases your vitality, makes you feel lighter and stronger, helps you to sustain your mental concentration, reduces the stresses on your immune system from the strains of everyday life, and empowers your energy levels. Establishing and maintaining an efficient lymphatic system can, therefore, help to increase the vigour and enthusiasm with which you approach sex.

Before we see how you can do this, let's look at what the lymphatic system is. To do so means first plunging back inside the body and immersing ourselves in one of its arteries. Carried along in the current created by the powerful rhythmic pulses of the heartbeat, we find our artery branching into smaller and ever smaller tributaries. At last we reach the finest of these, little more than the diameter of a blood cell. Here, the blood is forced by the irresistible tide of the heartbeat up against the capillary wall, pressing closer and closer to the soft lining tissue. As it touches this tissue, the nutrients and oxygen the blood has been carrying with it seep out from its cells and diffuse into the wall. It's almost as if the capillary wall were a filter.

As we watch these nutrients pass through the wall and out of sight, other material – waste products such as carbon dioxide, ammonia, mucus, and some dead cells – emerges into view through the capillary wall from whatever is on the other side. They are absorbed instantly by the blood. This deoxygenated blood then surges off, pulsing this time along a separate set of capillaries and into the veins. It recirculates through the kidneys (where it dumps the ammonia, used protein, excess minerals, and other impurities), the lungs (where it deposits the carbon dioxide and picks up more oxygen) before passing through the heart and surging once again into the arteries. The circulatory system, therefore, is a combined goods courier – a metabolic Federal Express – and waste-disposal operator.

But let's leave the endless cycles of the circulatory system behind and try to penetrate beyond the capillary wall. What is going on there, where do the nutrients and oxygen go and where do the waste products come from? Hanging onto a nutrient molecule as it passes through the capillary wall do we find ourselves in a muscle cell, perhaps, or a cell of soft connective tissue, part of a gland or an organ? No. Rather, we find ourselves dropping unceremoniously into a warm, salt-water ocean. This is called the interstitial fluid and to discover where this comes from means taking an even more mind-boggling journey of discovery, back to the Earth as it was at the dawn of time.

The Evolutionary Paddle

Life is thought to have begun in the mineral-rich oceans of our primordial world. Here, tiny single-cell organisms evolved using the suspended mineral solids around them to create the enzymes, proteins, and electrical currents they needed to power their existences. Living in such harmony with the water, they were, in effect, tiny specks of living water. Their cell walls were completely permeable, allowing the nutrients to flow through them, and from these nutrients they grew and reproduced.

Gradually, over millions and millions of years, the mineral content of the water dropped. One of nature's laws is that mineral concentrations must be equal in all parts of a liquid. This meant that to balance the concentrations, the organisms were forced to absorb so much water they burst and died. To compensate they started to evolve partly impermeable cell membranes. These would allow some nutrients to enter but would prevent too much water and other undesirable impurities from doing so. This process of selective entry is known as osmosis. Evolving this wall was one of the most decisive steps of all evolution. It effectively disengaged life from its completely harmonious coexistence with its environment. Since the organism could no longer simply flow away from its waste it evolved a crude waste-disposal tract, then lungs, a circulatory system, heart, kidneys, liver, and so on.

Today we are the dazzlingly complex results of this process of refinement and sophistication. You would imagine that we bore no relation to that primordial sea. But you would be wrong. For that sea is inside us. We evolved around it but our cells never learnt to live without it. While we now create machines that fly through space, and pose ourselves complex abstract questions about existence, each of us carries around 8 or 9 gallons of this primordial sea. And if you don't believe us, look what happens to you when you mildly burn yourself or scratch the surface of your skin: your skin doesn't bleed, it weeps. And in what environment can severed limbs or organs be kept alive? Salt water. What is sweat? Salt water. We need blood, certainly, but our cells feed directly from the water in the same way that those simple organisms did billions of years ago.

It is this water that makes up the lymphatic system. Sitting in the body in a fine, all-pervading mesh of tubes it acts as the interchange between the nutrient-carrying blood and the cells waiting to be fed. It swaps fresh oxygen and nutrients for carbon dioxide and waste products. It is this water-borne exchange that ensures firm, supple muscles that will neither tire easily nor cramp during exercise, unblemished skin, clear sparkling eyes, and shining hair. It ensures that you have stamina and energy, acute sensory perception, and a strong resistance to infection.

Currents of Health

The interstitial fluid of the lymphatic system is not an inert body of water. It is constantly moving and there is a very good reason for this. If you examine a small body of water, a garden pond perhaps, that is not fed by a replenishing supply of fresh water, it appears very stagnant. Rubbish accumulates on the bottom, moss gathers on the surface blocking out the light and killing the flora and fauna. If, on the other hand, this pond has a stream running through it, waste will not accumulate, the moss will be unable to gather, the water will be oxygenated, and life will flourish.

For much the same reasons, it is vital that the lymphatic fluid is constantly moving, passing around the body in the system's interconnecting tubules. This is because toxic waste products are emerging from the cells into the fluid, and must not be allowed to accumulate and block up the passages. Rather, they must be drained away from the cells and channelled into larger water-filled passages, finally arriving at the body's equivalent of sewage treatment works: the lymph nodes. Located in the groin, armpits and neck, these help to remove many of the impurities as well as producing antibodies, one of the body's first lines of defence against infection. (One of the giveaway symptoms of infection is a swelling of the nodes, clearly felt through the skin).

An efficiently flowing lymphatic system, therefore, is vitally important for a high level of vitality. However, don't forget that the system is the earliest remnant of our primordial, sea-borne past. Unlike the more recently evolved circulatory system, which is powered by means of a specifically designed organ, the heart, the lymph fluid has no power source. Rather, like an artesian well, it depends on pressure differentiation and the force of gravity to move it. Muscle contractions and relaxations, the continual opposition of large sets of muscles causing arms and legs to hinge, the spine to twist, and ribs to rise and fall, are vital for pushing the lymph fluid around the body. By alternately squeezing and releasing the lymphatic tubules that criss-cross the muscles in a fine mesh, they act like hydraulic bellows.

Exercise the Lymph

There are certain implications of this need to move the muscles. You may eat a superb diet of organic vegetables and freshly caught fish, leavened with pulses and wholemeal breads; you may supplement that diet with nutrients to help you counteract the pernicious effects of stress, anxiety, or depression; you might guard yourself against the combined health threats of smoking, alcohol, poor digestion, and the free radicals. However, if your lymphatic system isn't functioning healthily – if it becomes blocked with waste products – then all these measures may not prevent you from feeling sluggish, irritable, and easily fatigued, suffering from a puffy face, blotchy skin, joint pains, susceptibility to minor infection, a lack of stamina, and listlessness. The only way to make sure that the lymphatic system doesn't become blocked – the only way to sluice out the mucus and the broken proteins, the toxins, the specks of ammonia, and the agglomerations of fat – is to move those muscles. And the only way to do that is through exercise and deep breathing.

We realise that one of the most attractive aspects of using responsibly targeted and applied nutritional therapy is the ease with which you can do it. It may be a little inconvenient to swallow a few pills but, compared to some of the alternatives, it's child's play. However, the idea that simply by taking a few supplements and eating well you can ensure good health falters a little with the introduction of exercise into the equation. We know of nutritionists who have claimed in print that their only daily exercise is 30 seconds on a water bed but, by coupling this with a growth-hormone releasing pill, they can build up all the muscle they need. Unfortunately, for overall good health, there is no way of escaping it: you have to exercise. If you want to apply the tenets of this foundation course in vitality to move your sex life up a couple of gears, then you have to exercise. And the more vigorously and more often you do it, the more your muscles move and the greater will be the drainage of your lymphatic system.

What You Should Do

Like all animal species human beings have bodies that have been built for vigorous and sustained physical activity. With the agile, dextrous, upright stance, our forebears were ideally suited to meet the physical demands of hunting and gathering crops. In this active, itinerant life, their straining, working muscles were an ideal means of powering the lymphatic system.

Today, however, physique that was developed to help us in that prehistoric environment mostly goes to waste. We lead such sedentary lives. For a large proportion of the populace – including Dave, the man we met at the introduction to our vitality foundation course – the most physical activity they get is turning the steering wheel of their car. And, unfortunately, this inactivity is paid for with our health. Look around you, see how many people have sallow, puffy, blotchy skin, complain about aches and pains, suffer from regular infection, don't enjoy as vigorous and fulfilling a sex life as they would like. You might be one of them yourself. One of the main causes of these complaints must be the fact that their lymphatic systems are simply not draining adequately.

It is immensely important, therefore, to introduce some of the activity of our forebears into our own lives. Clearly, hunting for buffalo in Basingstoke is impractical, but there are a multitude of satisfactory exercises to choose from as alternatives: walking, jogging, running, stretching, skating, aerobics, yoga, cycling, swimming, tennis, squash, and badminton, to name a few.

One thing to bear in mind, though, is that the strenuousness of the exercise is not the most important factor involved in what you do (although it does play its part). As far as draining the lymphatic system is concerned, it is much more important that whatever exercise you decide to do is frequent. Three brisk half-hour walks a week, for example, will do you much more good than one intense, hour-long game of squash. If the exercise you choose is squash, therefore, it's important that you play at least three times a week or alternatively that you incorporate your single game into an exercise plan that includes other sports at other times of the week.

Whatever form of exercise you do take up, the key to making sure you continue doing it is that you enjoy it. For habitually sedentary people, the very idea of exercise can itself seem like an insurmountable obstacle, let alone actually getting down and doing it. If, once you start, you don't enjoy it, what better excuse could there be for giving up? If you're not used to exercise then whatever you do start slowly. If, for example, you decide to mix exercise with exploratory walks around your neighbourhood, try to set a pace of around four miles an hour. This is no sprint by any means, but it is a brisk, refreshing speed none the less. Furthermore, why confine yourself to the same exercise all the time? Walk one day, skip another; buy a miniature indoor trampoline and bounce around on it; go out for a swim; get on your bike. Mix it up and enjoy yourself. The changes to your life will be dramatic.

Building on the Foundation

So how can all the information we've looked at in the last three chapters be put to practical use in your own life? When it comes to laying the foundations for a deep and lasting vitality, which methods will suit you? Obviously the answer to this question will differ from person to person. It is very much a matter of feeling your way in, deciding what makes you feel good, and then sticking to it, resisting the temptation to slip back into old habits. To see just what can be achieved with these methods, let's meet our stressed sales manager, Dave, again, and see how the foundation course has changed his life.

It's a good four months after our last visit and he has already been applying many of the foundation-course precepts for ten weeks. We come upon him at 6.30 on a cold Monday morning with his alarm clock ringing. Instantly he is wide awake, feeling alert and refreshed rather than writhing semi-conscious under the duvet. He breathes deeply, gets up, does a series of gentle stretching exercises, then does ten chin-ups on the pull-up bar he has mounted on the bedroom doorframe. These exercises will not build up rippling sets of muscles, but what they will do is get the lymphatic system circulating to drain away any debris left over from the night and making everything clear for the fresh demands of nutrient distribution and waste disposal ahead.

Because his sleep is deeper and more invigorating he is able to sleep less. This means he can get up earlier and prepare a proper breakfast for himself and his wife, Rose. Rather than the previous unappetising meal of refined cereal coated in a frosting of sugar, they now eat a nutritious, delicious, and freshly made variation of a Swiss muesli recipe. Coming highly recommended by naturopaths this consists of a selection of chopped fruit (in this case apple, banana, and mango), several spoonfuls of porridge oats which have soaked in water overnight, organic yogurt which is naturally high in the benign bifidus bacteria cultures, honey, and a tablespoonful of freshly crushed linseeds.

This recipe sounds as if it must take hours to prepare and most people would argue that breakfast is the last meal where you want to spend any time slaving in the kitchen. However, in reality it takes no more than minutes to prepare and is so much better for you than either toast and cereal or a 'traditional' cooked breakfast. Just look at its advantages: the fresh fruit is rich not only in vitamins and minerals but also in natural enzymes that will help the gut with digestion; the oats, which after their soaking have already started the breakdown of their complex carbohydrate forms into simpler and more easily digested forms, will provide some bulk and fibre; the yogurt will help with digestion, supply calcium and many important B vitamins, and increase the transit time of the food; and the crushed linseeds will provide a natural, easily assimilated source of two essential polyunsaturated fatty acids. Not only is this mixture of fruit, honey, oats, and grains delicious and full of nutrition, therefore, it will actually work with the body's digestive system rather than against it.

At the same time Dave takes dietary supplements of vitamins A, C, and E to, among other things, protect himself from the effects of free radicals. He also takes a supplement of phenylalanine to empower him to thrive on the stresses of the day ahead.

However, Dave still has to endure the traumatic and infuriating drive to work. He arrives feeling a little ragged but resists the temptation to take his coffee machine from the bottom drawer of his filing cabinet where it has sat for the last six weeks. This afternoon he has a meeting with the board to set budgets for the next financial year and he anticipates a difficult time. Conscious of a sense of anxiety in his stomach, he works steadily on his board presentation throughout the morning. However, rather than pressing on regardless when his concentration flags, he stands up, stretches then lays out the mini-trampoline he has bought for just this purpose on his office floor. Then, for five minutes, he pounds up and down on it for all he is worth. This procedure is repeated every 45 minutes or so throughout the morning and each time he returns to his work he finds his concentration vastly improved.

At lunchtime he puts down his pen and goes out for a short, brisk walk, pausing every now and then to look in a shop window or browse in a newsagent. He reaches a health-food restaurant where he orders a plate of salad crammed with pulses, high in protein, and bean shoots. A supplement of glutamic acid is taken with the salad, then it's back to work.

At the board meeting he is calm, lucid, and confident. He even has time to look at the faces of his colleagues and is startled to recognise in them the telltale signs of anxiety once such a familiar sight in the mirror: they appear witty and animated but the pallid, sallow skin, the eyes ringed by blue diaphanous smudges, and the corners of their eyes and nostrils pink with a suggestion of rawness are unmistakable. Everyone gulps down coffee except Dave, who is pointedly drinking uncarbonated mineral water.

His whole working day is now a highly successful exercise in stress diversion and management. He can cope much more productively with the demands on his energy and, when the pangs of anxiety do start to bite, he is prepared to use them nutritionally to his advantage. In this way the stresses that once blighted his waking life have become tools to help him enjoy it.

Since Dave now works so much more productively, he is able to leave work at a sane time and even fits in a hard-fought game of squash. He gets home at about the same time as Rose and together they cook a meal of poached salmon, salad, and baked potatoes.

Dave's new routines may sound very dull and precious. A lot of readers may find his life more interesting the way it was before: its unpredictability, its peaks and troughs of emotion, the constant, energy-sapping need to live on his nerves. That life has something of an adventure about it. On the other hand, if you want to look for real adventure, then look no further than Dave and Rose's revitalised sex life. The change in routine – the lymphatic drainage exercises, the stress management, the responsible approach to nutritional supplementation, and the diversity of good, nutrient-rich foods – have helped to transform it out of all recognition.

For them both it's as if the level of their emotional intensity and their libido has shifted up several gears. Sometimes when they're in bed together Dave feels saturated with energy and wellbeing. He is much stronger now, is much more aware of the delights of using his body, and makes love with a passion, vigour, determination, and joy that he has never before experienced. And their sex is so much more varied. Now they are inquisitive about how much pleasure they can give. They change the pace of their lovemaking, massage each other, enjoying the sheer physical exertion of their straining muscles, taking great gulps of air and laughing.

Summary

We cannot underestimate the importance of ensuring that your body eliminates efficiently the toxic waste products of the metabolic pathways. Effective elimination is essential for a strong immune system, extended stamina, pliant muscles, clear skin, and high energy levels. Aerobic exercise for at least 30 minutes three times a week is therefore a vital component of the good-sex foundation that we have built.

Part 3
The Good Sex Nutrition Programme

It would be wonderful to say: 'Here is a pill. Pop one in your mouth every day and it will cure all your sexual problems. It will allow you to make love for longer, increase your feelings of pleasure, intensify your orgasm, and raise your stamina levels so that you can make love over and over and over again.'

Unfortunately we can't do that. The human sexual response is one of the most complicated processes of interrelating metabolic pathways that exists. It requires the presence of many raw-material nutrients, each of which is important to the use the body makes of the others. Only by supplying a selection of those nutrients implicated in the sex response is it possible to effect changes.

This multiple use of nutrients is called synergy. In the past few years, the word 'synergy' has been much used to denote the way in which different parties – copywriter and visualiser, brewer and food company – complement each other when brought together, each enhancing the attributes of the other. Exactly the same holds true for nutritional supplementation. To elicit the desired sexual responses means providing the metabolic pathways with groups of nutrients that create metabolic synergy: overlapping, complementing, empowering, and intensifying. To this end, the following chapters will carry sometimes quite long lists of nutrients for treating particular complaints, be it low stamina, premature ejaculation, frigidity, lack of physical sensations, or dry vagina. Faced with the prospect of perhaps on occasion having to take several supplements at once over a period of weeks or even months, you might feel tempted to give up. If so, all we can say is don't. The supplement programme in this book represents a thorough, comprehensive, synergistic selection of nutrients designed to improve your sexuality at the deepest level. Used carefully they can work for you.

Chapter 6

The Best-Kept Sex Secret in the World

We've now seen how important the general health and wellbeing of your body is for achieving good sex. We've also looked at ways of reaching this height of vitality. The guidelines covered in the last five chapters are, out of necessity, brief summaries of very complex subjects. Entire books have been written about issues we could only touch on in a paragraph. (If you are interested in further reading, a bibliography is included at the back of this book.) What the previous chapters have done is to show you ways of laying a foundation of general vitality.

Assuming that you are clear about the importance of this 'foundation', it's now time to focus our attention on specific sexual matters. Throughout the rest of the book, therefore, we'll unravel the origins of many of the most common causes of sexual anxiety, frustration, and disappointment. We'll deal with, among others, premature ejaculation, impotence, frigidity, lack of physical sensations, low sperm count, and dry vaginal walls. Understanding some of the causes will in turn help to show which nutrients are needed to help alleviate which problems. Much of this advice may prove to be useful even if you already enjoy a healthy sex life. It simply means that by following the nutritional guidelines you'll be making things even better than they are already.

So let's start by looking at the intimate role the chemical histamine plays in assisting with ejaculation and orgasm.

The Jekyll and Hyde Chemical

Histamine is created in one of the body's metabolic pathways from its parent molecule, histidine. Found naturally in food sources such as cereals, histidine straddles a grey borderline between being seen as a dietary essential (meaning that it cannot be manufactured in the body from other substances) and non-essential amino acid. Like all aminos, histidine is a highly versatile molecule and is used for a variety of purposes in the blood stream and by the cells. It is known to encourage the secretion of digestive gastric juices, particularly stomach acid. And it is a good chelator. This means that when ingested by the body in controlled amounts it can latch onto, and eject, heavy metal toxins such as cadmium, mercury, and lead.

Histidine is also an important inhibitory neurotransmitter. When secreted by the axons into the synaptic voids which separate one cell from the next, it generates calming alpha-wave-inducing brain messages. For this reason it is a natural tranquilliser and one of the body's inbuilt counterbalances to excitory neurotransmitters such as adrenalin. In fact, low histidine levels have been found to contribute to a number of psychological disorders ranging from lethargy, fatigue, poor appetite, and nausea through to serious problems such as anxiety neurosis and schizophrenia. Because of this, some health professionals actually recommend histidine as part of an amino acid anxiety-neutralising formula.

Although these are all vital biological functions, what concerns us more are the reactions that occur once this calm, soothing, Dr Jekyll-type molecule, histidine, is converted into histamine, an unruly, brawling, uncontrollable Mr Hyde. For while we associate histidine with mental tranquillity, histamine has quite different functions: as well as fighting infection it is also one of the causes of ejaculation and orgasm. How histamine causes these reactions is what we'll look at next.

The Boiling-Oil Molecule

Histamine is a central component of the body's immune response. It battles biological invaders such as viruses, bacteria, environmental toxins, and allergens. As soon as any of these invaders start to affect the body's tissue, certain organelles called mast cells burst, inundating them in histamine the way the defenders of a castle would pour boiling oil on a siege army. In turn, this sudden histamine deluge has the effect of stimulating production of a group of substances called T-helper cells. These are rapid-response bodies produced in the thymus gland (hence their T prefix) which break down and neutralise attackers. A telltale sign of T-cell activity against infection is swelling, redness, inflammation, congestion, and rashes around the affected area.

Since the histamine is the source of this inflammation, an excess of the chemical will encourage extra T-cell production, regardless of whether a cause of infection is present or not. This means that the body will react with those same characteristic symptoms of redness, swelling, itching, and so on, but for no obvious cause. And this response will be aggravated by the fact that histamine also makes the capillaries dilate, causing blood to suffuse through the skin and leading to an uncomfortable, prickly redness. These symptoms of histamine excess are closely linked with allergies. An allergy is, after all, an immune response to basically harmless substances such as pollen, cat fur, and gluten. It is also the reason why anti-histamines are often prescribed to combat such allergic reactions.

This histamine-generated response gives us a clear insight into the mechanism which causes orgasm and ejaculation. Masters and Johnson documented a clear connection between the histamine-derived immune response and reactions that occur at the time of orgasm. This was confirmed in publications such as the *American Medical Journal* and *Human Sexuality*, which observed that common responses during sex – such as a reddening of the skin, hives, salivation, sneezing, asthma, chills, and shivering – were identical to the immune response. And the common thread appeared to be histamine.

Further research revealed that histamine-containing mast cells are highly concentrated in the glans (or head) of the penis and throughout the clitoris. And Carl Pfeiffer, one of America's most respected experts in the field of nutrition and health, observed how these particular mast cells release histamine immediately before orgasm. This, he suggested, was a key factor both in orgasm itself and the minute spasms of ejaculation that occur a moment later. It seems faintly absurd to compare orgasm to an immune response, but the mechanism is quite similar. However, if excess histamine leads to allergies – that is, immune responses to non-existent threats – what does histamine do for the sexual response? Cause premature ejaculation, perhaps?

Following this line of questioning, Pfeiffer realised that if, as seemed likely, a healthy level of blood and tissue histamine determined orgasm and ejaculation, then higher or lower levels would cause a change in those conditions. Higher than average levels of histamine would indeed trigger orgasm and ejaculation prematurely, while lower histamine would indeed trigger orgasm and ejaculation prematurely, while lower histamine levels might even prevent orgasm from occurring at all, prolonging the lovemaking to the point where it became painful and arousal disappeared. Obviously, Pfeiffer's findings have major implications for both male and female. Let's first see how they can be used to help female sexuality.

Breaking Down the Barrier

A surprisingly large number of women are unable to reach orgasm. There are many different reasons for this. Stress at work or at home, tension with a partner, a variety of conditions which prevent relaxation. Perhaps the lover is unable or unwilling to provide sufficient stimulation. He may achieve orgasm long before she does, a common occurrence, then inconsiderately turn over and fall asleep rather than helping to ensure that his partner is satisfied. Then again, some women, despite a supportive and loving environment, are physically unable to orgasm. They may well be barred the intense physical sensations and stimulation of intercourse as well as the climax itself. This state is unkindly called frigidity, an unhelpful catch-all word that only serves to make sufferers feel more wretched and inadequate, reinforcing as it does a picture of cold brittleness.

However, hope is at hand for, as Carl Pfeiffer has discovered, this inability may well be related to low levels of histamine. If so, then supplementing the diet with histadine (the parent molecule of histamine) could prove to be the means of a wonderful release from the problem. The evidence for the effects of histadine/histamine is by no means conclusive, but Pfeiffer's work makes a compelling argument in its favour. As long ago as the mid-1970s he conducted a study on a large group of women volunteers, all of whom suffered from an inability to orgasm. During his tests he found that, in tandem with their sexual problems, most of these women had suffered for some time from psychological difficulties. These included depression and anxiety and ranged considerably in their degree of severity.

It is not clear whether such problems were caused by the frigidity or that they actually caused it. Whichever was the case it was certain that their unstable mental states were contributing to poor and insufficient nutritional intake. Stress and anxiety, after all, rapidly deplete the body of essential nutrients and can trigger a downward spiral of increasingly inadequate supplies of raw materials to the body's metabolic pathways. Furthermore, since histidine acts as an inhibitory neurotransmitter, a lack of this chemical would contribute to their susceptibility to anxiety and stress. Pfeiffer couldn't have been surprised when, with further testing, he found that a large proportion of the women in his study group showed histidine levels far below the norm.

To counter the effects of their poor nutrition he devised diets high in every essential nutrient. Then, to test his theories about the correlation between low histidine levels and an inability to orgasm, he began introducing histidine supplements into their diets. On average he administered a 500 mg dose of the amino acid before each meal. A large proportion of his study group subsequently reported an alleviation, and in some cases even disappearance, of their symptoms. Not only did they find that orgasm was much easier to achieve, but that the physical intensity and pleasure experienced during sex was much greater. Since the histidine supplements would probably have had a calming effect as well, this might help to account for their reactions. Many of these women, after all, suffered from anxiety, stress, and other tensions, all of which must have interfered with the delicate see-saw, excitation/relaxation nature of sex.

Of course, it's not only women who will benefit from histidine supplementation. Some men, while achieving penile erection, are similarly unable to reach a climax. A lack of histamine in the mast cells of the glans seems one of the most likely causes and, indeed, the problem has been treated with great success by some nutritionists using supplements of histidine.

If you feel you would like to use histidine supplements start with small infrequent doses – perhaps 500 mg a day with meals – and slowly increase the amount if necessary. It's a good idea to be a little cautious since some women have found that amounts higher than 4 grams a day can bring on their menstrual cycles prematurely. Indeed, women athletes have been known to take doses of histidine in excess of 4 grams to ensure that their periods do not coincide with important sporting competitions. Finally, to help the histidine change to histamine, it's a good idea to take co-factor supplements of vitamins B3 and B6.

Beating Premature Ejaculation

Of course, it's a good deal easier to raise a person's blood and tissue levels of histamine than it is to lower them. However, this is just what has to happen if a man wants to tackle one of the most likely causes of premature ejaculation: excess histamine in the blood and mast cells. Like the stigma of frigidity, premature ejaculation can be no laughing matter. For some men, ejaculation can be caused simply by engaging in foreplay or hugging, or even watching sex on screen or reading about it in a magazine or book. Even in the most sensitive and supportive relationships it can, if the problem continues, create severe, divisive strains between partners. It can engender a sense of humiliation and frustration, a feeling of not being in control of your body. In such circumstances it's difficult not to feel sorry for yourself or to experience extra tension during sexual encounters caused by the possibility of failure.

Excess histamine is no more the sole cause of premature ejaculation than a deficiency is the cause of an inability to orgasm. None the less, there is every suggestion that it does play a significant role. So how do you go about lowering the body's histamine levels? Firstly, it's not a matter of simply excluding histidine-rich foods from the diet. Although histidine is present in its highest concentrations in cereals, it can be found in all proteinous foods. Even if you were able to pinpoint those foods so precisely that your intake dropped, it is likely that your body would be able to manufacture it from other amino acids. However, in doing so it could well drain the metabolic pathways of nutrients – enzymes, co-factors, and amino acids – that would be better employed elsewhere.

So what other means are there for lowering these recalcitrant histamine levels? The answer lies with some quite separate research Pfeiffer conducted into the nutrient levels of schizophrenic patients. During this research he found that their blood-histamine levels were inordinately high. Whether the schizophrenia was caused by an overburdening of the brain cells with the inhibitory histidine is not clear. However, in his search for means of reducing the almost stratospherically high histamine levels he came across the effects of the amino acid methionine.

Unlike histidine, methionine is recognisably an essential amino. It is also one of a group of four so-called sulphur-based amino acids. What this means is that in addition to the atoms of oxygen, hydrogen, and carbon, which come as standard with all amino acids, it also has an optional extra in the form of a sulphur atom. We tend to think of sulphur as an airborne pollutant, disgorged in billowing plumes from power stations. Yet in our bodies it is a vital component of healthy skin, bones, organs, and hair. Because of its sulphur atom, methionine is recognised as a beauty supplement. It is used to increase the tone, elasticity, and vigour of skin. It can add sheen and bounce to hair and strengthen nails that have a tendency to split, giving them a robust tensile quality rather than the brittleness obtained from lacquering.

More to the point, methionine, a main component, must be activated before it is effective. When activated it is called s-adenosyl methionine. This is a particularly active component of the metabolic pathways, causing numerous chemical reactions. It brings different chemicals together like a tireless society hostess introducing party guests whom she thinks might get on. In addition to the methionine itself, several co-factors are needed to create s-adenosyl methionine. In particular these are the minerals calcium and magnesium and the vitamins B1 and B3.

What would our diplomatic party hostess do if her soirée were crashed by a noisy, insulting, uninvited stranger? Rather than allowing him to disrupt the party she would, as diplomatically and unostentatiously as possible, usher him into a quiet ante-room. At the same time, a discrete hand signal would draw the attention of a couple of burly attendants to hurl the trouble-maker into the street. This is, more or less, how s-adenosyl methionine works. Not only does it divert excess histamine from those reactions where it can cause the most mischief, it is also a catalyst in the creation of one of the body's burliest bouncers: the excitory neurotransmitter, adrenalin. This has a mediating function on histamine, helping to offset the effects of excessively high histamine levels.

To Pfeiffer's undoubted satisfaction, the administration of methionine with its enzyme-creating co-factors helped to relieve many of the symptoms of schizophrenia in his patients. Taking his findings a stage further, it was a natural progression to examine the effects of this therapy on victims of premature ejaculation caused by high levels of histamine. Administered in the same way, the supplements had the effect in a large number of his patients of increasing the time it took them to achieve orgasm and ejaculate. Imagine their sense of relief and liberation!

Gut Reactions

Another suspected cause of excess blood-histamine levels can be traced to the gut. You may remember that in chapter 4 we looked at the effects of poor digestion. One of the consequences was that much of the undigested food tends to putrefy in the gut, releasing potential toxins such as octopamine, which can interfere with the neurotransmitters, and even, in extreme cases, nitrosamines, which may cause cancer. Another product of putrefaction is histamine. Seeping into the blood through the gut lining, it is thought that it will then interfere with the body's immune response as well as contributing to premature ejaculation.

Any attempt at reducing excess histamine levels should therefore include a programme of measures to improve your digestion. These include the amino-acid complex to stimulate digestive enzymes, and plenty of raw foods and salads to assist the enzymes in their functions. You should also include in your diet high-fibre foods such as pulses and fruits to help speed up the passage of food through the bowel, assisted by fatty foods such as fish and unadultered oils. You will find the details of this programme in Chapter 4. And hopefully it will help to explain while the foundation course in vitality is so important. There can't be many people who would think that poor digestion can have a bearing on premature ejaculation.

His and Her Histidine

Apart from the work conducted by Carl Pfeiffer there has been precious little scientific analysis of the effects of histidine and histamine on sexual experience. However, what is certain from numerous practical accounts is that it has been used by nutritional therapists to enhance the lives of hundreds of people suffering from unsatisfactory sexual responses. Used wisely, it can help to unblock the feelings of repression and inadequacy, anger and guilt experienced by those who otherwise feel barred from expressing themselves sexually. Equally, an awareness of the potential ramifications of histamine excess can help to increase the sexual longevity and satisfaction of many men. With so few published findings into their effects, it is hardly surprising that the benefits of histamine and methionine are known only to a select few. Because of this it must be one of the best-kept sex secrets of the century.

To illustrate just how potent histamine therapy can be, let's look at a couple of case histories.

Adelle is a woman in her late thirties. A little over two years ago she and her husband separated and she moved in with another man, Tom. Despite the best intentions, the separation generated into a free-for-all of acrimony and recrimination. Having left her two teenage children with her husband, Adelle was made to feel irresponsible, selfish, and cruel for leaving, while he did all he could to make access to them difficult. Having also disaffected many of her former friends by the separation, with no one apart from Tom to confide in, she started to suffer from a heady mixture of anxiety, self-loathing, and depression. She ate little and suffered from severe insomnia. 'I think,' she concedes, 'that I might have become anorexic.'

Unsurprisingly, life with her lover became difficult. He found her quiet and listless. At times, dwelling on the turmoil of her life, she would suffer a near-hysterical anxiety attack, and Tom's attempts to soothe her would, in turn, lead to blazing rows. Sexually, their relationship was very unsatisfying. She felt little interest in making love and, on those rare occasions when they did attempt to do so, she experienced no sensation of pleasure, and was unable either to climax or return any of Tom's passion.

'Everything was wretched. He blamed himself for my state while I looked at the way things had reached this rock-bottom level as a kind of retribution for what I'd done, the way I'd treated my kids. I felt I deserved to suffer.' However, help was at hand in the form of nutritional supplementation. Following a nutritional counselling session, she started using a complex of amino acids – phenylalanine to add mental energy and enthusiasm, and histidine, to stimulate the calming alpha-wave-generating neurotransmitters and to help her with her lack of sexual response – taken together with the co-factors of copper, magnesium, vitamins B3, B6, C, and folic acid. 'After this things took a turn for the better,' she says. In terms of her emotions, she reported more zest for life and more fortitude in facing up to her problems. Furthermore, probably thanks to the help of the histidine, she is starting to enjoy the physical side of her relationship with Tom once more.

At the other end of the spectrum is Brian, a man in his early thirties who has suffered from premature ejaculation since his first sexual encounter in his mid-teens. 'I've had some incredibly humiliating experiences,' he recalls. 'It was worse when I was younger because you feel everything very intensely and I couldn't put any sense of perspective on things. I suffered agonies then, even though the girls with whom it happened were on the whole quite understanding. You can't believe the heart-rending, tantalising sense of hopelessness I'd experience. To be so close, to really want to do it, then, with sinking heart, to feel everything happen too fast, slipping out of control, and it would be over and I'd feel rotten. My doctor was pretty insensitive and said that it was a common aspect of growing up, that it was all in my mind and that I would get over it. I remember thinking then, "How is it going to change?" '

Admittedly, as Brian got older, the severity of his problem lessened and sex became possible. 'It was still a fairly short-lived thing, though, I'm sorry to say. It meant I developed an acrobatic line in foreplay but, no matter how good that was, it wasn't the real thing.'

Brian's first inkling that nutritional supplementation could help came from browsing through a previous book of ours, *The Amino Revolution*, in a bookshop. Intrigued by the possibilities, he made an appointment for a counselling session. One of the points that surfaced very quickly from the consultation was that his skin marked very easily; the slightest pressure would provoke red patches. Likewise, the rims of his eyes were often red and irritable, suggesting a mild allergy even though, as far as he knew, he was not allergic to anything. These signs pointed to blood and cellular histamine levels above the norm and subsequent testing confirmed this. Accordingly, it was suggested that Brian take supplemental methionine together with co-factors vitamins B3, B6, folic acid, and C, magnesium and calcium. He was also recommended the amino-acid complex to improve the production of digestive enzymes and given a list of fibre and enzyme-rich raw foods to increase the speed of passage.

Another Best-Kept Secret
Finally, he was given an exercise to try that a number of patients with similar problems had found effective in the past: namely, rather than moving his penis in and out of his girlfriend's vagina as usual – and incurring the customary premature ejaculation from stimulating histamine release from the glans – he was to keep it fully inserted. He was then alternately to clench and relax his buttocks. This would have the effect of pushing his pelvic bone up against her clitoris. The result would be that the clitoris would continue to be stimulated while at the same time minimising stimulation of the penis glans, thereby increasing longevity. Hopefully, everyone ends up a good deal more satisfied.

Happily, both technique and the supplementation seemed to work very well. Brian is able to make love for much longer periods. 'It's great because I can relax into it and enjoy it and not have to be sort of constantly on the look out and dreading that moment when I ejaculate. Even now I can still feel it happening sooner than I want but with that little technique I can stave it off that much more. I realise now that this problem was giving me a guilt complex as well as everything else; I felt I was taking more from my partner than I was giving her. It's wonderful to know that now I can give her as much satisfaction and pleasure as she gives me.'

Summary

Excessive body levels of the amino-acid derivative, histamine, are a cause of premature ejaculation. Lower-than-average levels often contribute to frigidity. For men wishing to reduce their histamine levels we recommend:

1 A mixture of the amino acid methionine together with co-factors calcium, magnesium, B3, B6, folic acid, and C.
2 A programme designed to improve digestion and including the complete amino-acid blend, fresh fruits and vegetables, high-fibre foods, fish, and fatty acids.

Women who experience difficulty reaching orgasm should try a supplement of histamine's parent molecule, histidine, together with co-factors copper, magnesium, B3, B6, C, and folic acid.

Chapter 7
Energising Your Sex Life

In this chapter we're going to look at ways of increasing the energy you have for sex. With more energy, lovemaking becomes increasingly exciting and the means of exploring each other's sexuality more varied and prolonged. More energy creates stronger desire and deeper passion and this in turn is reflected in the vigour with which you make love.

Although to a certain extent the energy expended in lovemaking, and the resulting physical excitation and arousal, depends on how much adrenalin is circulating, it is also related to the body's fundamental ability to burn and release fuel. In this sense it is similar to the carburettor of your car. You might fill the tank with the highest octane petrol, but if the carburettor is clogged then the fuel will not be allowed to combust efficiently and the performance of the car will suffer. As with your car, so with your body. For many people their energy-liberating systems – their cellular carburettors – do not operate as well as they should. This means that they tire easily, that they are physically weak, and that they will be unable to sustain periods of physical stimulation. And as far as sex is concerned it will lead to a lack of, or an inability to sustain, arousal during lovemaking.

This is a common problem for both sexes but for men especially. It sometimes causes men's penises to go limp for no apparent reason during sex and robs them of sexual desire. We have spoken to several men who have described how, during sexual encounters, their sex drive seems to desert them. One man, Nigel, conjured the image of his libido running on a strictly rationed meter that may expire at any moment.

'I was alone for the first time with a woman I'd desired for some months. She had invited me to her flat for dinner and, late in the evening, asked me if I wanted to stay the night. I said yes, experiencing a mixture of relief and desire, yet, when we went to bed, I felt curiously unemotional and unattached about the whole thing. We fumbled around in bed. We engaged in foreplay but I simply couldn't get an erection. Here I was with this lovely, intelligent, desirable lady and I felt washed out and impotent.'

'My problem,' says another man, called Jamie, 'is that sometimes after penetration I lose my erection and I feel empty and passionless inside. I don't think it's anything to do with my wife as, after six years of marriage, I still find her as gorgeous as the day I first saw her. Unfortunately she thinks that I don't fancy her any more and, as the proof of the pudding is in the eating, the physical signs probably confirm this.'

And women, too, describe similar experiences of how a lack of energy spoils their lovemaking. Sybil, for example:

'Sometimes when we make love my husband asks me to respond more and he worries that my lack of demonstrativeness is a reflection of inability on his part to please me. It's not that at all, it's just that sometimes I don't feel like responding. It takes too much effort and I simply can't be bothered to lift myself up. I'm not cold to him and he does arouse me, but I just can't be bothered.'

What follows are a selection of nutritional supplements unparalleled for their ability to unleash the energy stored in every cell of your body. Used wisely these supplements can energise your sex life, making it more active, exciting and fulfilling, increasing your strength and endurance and completely overcoming any problems of lack of arousal.

The Yin and Yang of Sexual Energy

Chinese philosophers believe that life is made up of two fundamentally opposing forces. Called yin and yang they are symbolised as two shapes – fish perhaps, or teardrops, or possibly even sperm – interlocking to form a perfect circle. Yin and yang represent light and darkness, life and death, attack and retreat, push and pull, man and woman, sperm and egg. Most importantly, they represent creation and destruction. Eschewing our modern-day perceptions of one being positive and the other negative, the Chinese saw these two forces as individually essential for the survival of the other, like an eternally ebbing and flowing tide. As with so much of what the ancient philosophers wrote about, yin and yang are a perfect way of representing in metaphor the never-ending tidal forces within the body. For the body's ability to use and release energy is wholly dependent on a metabolic yin and yang.

Biochemically, yin and yang are similar to the body's anabolic and catabolic phases. You may have heard of the term anabolic in connection with the banned steroid substances used by athletes to create greater muscle bulk. Simply, anabolic means to build up, and all the building processes in the body – be it assembling muscle protein, stimulating cell division, or generating enzymes – are anabolic, as are all the chemical processes that involve the creation or reproduction of one substance from another, simpler substance. Because this is a creative, building process, all anabolic activities consume energy. It needs considerable energy, after all, to bond many different chemicals together, and that energy is stored, latent and unusable, in those bonds.

Catabolic activity, on the other hand, is closely linked with the breaking down of these substances. Catabolic activity tears tissue apart, destroys enzymes and cells and strips protein structures like a written-off car being stripped of parts in a scrap-yard. And, by tearing those substances apart and thereby obliterating those bonds which created them, this process frees large quantities of energy, releasing it for other uses. While the anabolic phase is a measured application of order, therefore, the catabolic phase signifies the chaotic supremacy of anarchy. And all this carrying on in your body.

You may imagine from this that the anabolic phase, the yin of the body, is a good, positive, creative aspect of life, while the catabolic is destructive and wasteful. The truth is that each needs the other. The anabolic phase, for example, encourages the growth of certain illnesses which flourish in an environment that nurtures a building up of structures. Viruses such as herpes, encephalitis, influenza, and glandular fever love being in an anabolic environment. So does cancer. It is the body's catabolic phase, its tendency to tear things down, which protects it from these threats before they have a chance to hurt it. On the other hand, the putrefaction of food is also a catabolic activity.

Much of the investigative work in this area was conducted by the pioneering doctor Emmanuel Revici. He discovered that every vitamin, mineral, amino acid, and fatty acid, and indeed every food, was either anabolic or catabolic and that eating more of one or the other variety can actually help to tilt the body's balance between these two phases. While most amino acids encourage the building up of protein structures and are therefore anabolic, there is a small group of aminos that have the opposite effect. Revici suggested that by using one or other of these groups of foods it should be possible to offset the effects of anabolically or catabolically based disorders. If, for example, someone suffered from a virus infection – an anabolic response – it should be possible by increasing the intake of specifically identified catabolic foods to break the virus down.

Breaking Open Your Energy

Now, as we've seen, the anabolic phase of your body consumes energy while catabolic activity liberates energy. By taking supplements, therefore, that stimulate the catabolic functioning of the body, you can actually help to unleash reserves of energy that previously lay dormant within the cells. The catabolic amino acids which can help this to happen are methionine, taurine, cysteine, asparagine, and glutamic acid, and together they can make a potent energy-raising formula.

The best time of day for taking this catabolic formula is between 4 and 10 p.m. This period coincides with the phase when the body's own natural catabolic activity is at its height, as opposed to the six hours between 4 and 10 a.m. when the building-up, anabolic, reactions take place. Try taking the catabolic supplements with your evening meal. In following these guidelines some people have remarked how the resulting increase in energy has physically galvanised them. 'I feel all charged up,' said one young woman after coming for nutritional counselling. 'I could concentrate more easily, my limbs and muscles felt more pliant, and when my boyfriend and I make love it's better than ever it was because we're so much more active and playful and adventurous and intense all at the same time.'

The Metabolic Engineer

Another amino acid which is closely linked with energy release is carnitine. This is a combination of two amino acids, lysine and methionine, which are brought together in the liver. Its energy-releasing potential is so great that you should consider taking it as a supplement in its own right (although do make sure that you take the l-carnitine form and not the dl-carnitine). Here's why.

Simply, l-carnitine has an immensely important function as a carrier molecule. In common with many other amino acids, it is used by the body to ferry raw-material substances around the body like a molecular taxi. Fleets of amino acids, for example, are used to pick up freshly digested food molecules in the gut then transport them safely across the gut lining into the blood stream. You may have had first-hand experience of the job amino acids do in carrying molecules around if you take a mineral supplement. Many such supplements are 'chelated' to make them more bio-available. Often, this means that an amino acid has been used to latch onto the mineral molecule like a claw to give it a piggy-back into the body. While other molecules do act as chelators, we believe that amino acids are the best.

The carrier role that particularly interests us, though, takes place not in the gut or the blood stream but deep inside the oceanic expanse of the cell interior. Carnitine is such an important molecule for energy release because it conveys fatty-acid molecules through the cytoplasmic depths of the cell to tiny organelles called mitochondria. Mitochondria, the cell's furnaces, are one of the means used by the body to create energy for the chemical reactions of life. Here the fatty acid is carried across the mitochondria wall then, in the presence of oxygen, is burnt, combusted in an instantaneous microscopic flash to release energy.

Carnitine's involvement in this can be compared to that of an engineer on the footplate of a steam train. His job is to feed the train's furnace by shovelling hundredweight after hundredweight of coal into the furnace to generate the heat that will in turn create the steam for powering the engine's wheels. If insufficient coal is shovelled into the furnace there will not be enough energy to move the train. In the same way, a lack of carnitine will lead to lower energy levels. This will not only enervate your body, it may also lead to a build-up of fat and cholesterol in the blood and in the cells. Likewise, it can encourage ketosis, an accumulation of tarry waste products that make the blood more acidic and consequently cause it to dump acid-sensitive minerals such as calcium, magnesium, potassium, and zinc into the urine.

Because of its effect on fat levels, carnitine is used both by slimmers to reduce weight and by victims of cardiovascular disorders to provide energy and to reduce their blood cholesterol levels. More relevant for us, though, the respected health author Leslie Kenton reports how it is used widely by athletes for its ability to increase the level of energy by having the fatty acids burnt. Consequently, she says, it raises stamina and endurance and, in animal experiments, it has even been found to lengthen lifespan. It is usually taken up to six times a day as a 250 mg capsule on an empty stomach. One note of caution: since increasing your carnitine levels may also raise the amount of fat in the cells waiting to be oxidised, it could encourage the problems of rancidity associated with free-radical activity that we examined in Chapter 4. For this reason it is best taken with the antioxidant nutrients vitamins C and E.

Grow Your Own Energy

One further selection of energy-producing amino acids worth considering is a group which stimulates secretion of an important chemical called somatrophic hormone, otherwise known as growth hormone. Growth hormone is secreted by the pituitary gland to control the rate at which protein structures are manufactured from their raw-material-nutrient components. It stimulates firm, supple muscle growth, the formation of long bones, clear, healthy skin, and strong organs. And, in common with carnitine, it inhibits excess fat formation by mobilising fatty acids to be burnt for energy. Growth hormone production is highest in growing children, hence their ability to eat vast amounts of food without getting fat. It is also found in levels much higher than average in the blood of athletes. This is probably due to the fact that their strenuous physical exercise saturates their cells with oxygen and this is itself a growth-hormone release stimulant. This helps to explain why their muscle tone is so much more developed than normal, and why their stamina, strength and energy reserves run much deeper.

For most people, growth-hormone release declines sharply after the age of 30 and this is thought to be one of the causes of the muscle wastage and bone thinning that occurs as we enter middle age. For most people beyond their mid-thirties, the available growth hormone is used simply to carry out the necessary running repairs on the body: healing wounds, regenerating wasted cells, resisting infection by stimulating immune-system activity, and so on. And the lack of additional growth hormone means that energy levels may decrease while fat deposits are allowed to accumulate in the blood vessels, soft tissue, and cells.

However, this rather fatalistic view of growth-hormone loss is now known to be misplaced. Whatever your age, whether 20 or 60, there are ways of actually increasing your body's levels of growth hormone. One of these is to exercise regularly. As we saw in chapter 5, exercise is vital for ensuring an efficient drainage of your lymphatic system. As collateral, such exercise, assuming it is aerobic (that is, involves breathing hard and therefore increasing the cellular oxygen levels), will also stimulate the secretion of growth hormone, helping your muscles to remain firm and pliant, your skin to stay youthful and the blood-fat and blood-cholesterol levels to stay low. Paradoxically, therefore, up to a certain point, the more exercise you do, and the more strenuous it becomes, the higher your energy levels will climb.

Furthermore, this growth-hormone release can be complimented by using certain amino acids which stimulate the pituitary into secreting additional growth hormone. The aminos in question are arginine and lysine. With their help new muscle protein will be created, the tensile strength of structural protein increased and, perhaps most importantly, the fat deposits will release free fatty acids into the blood stream, there to be burnt both by the liver and by the mitochondria to release energy.

Arginine has many other uses in the body. It helps to detoxify ammonia, regulates the body's nitrogen balance and encourages semen production (of which we'll see more in chapter 9). Since it is used so widely, shortages may occur if the diet isn't as balanced as it should be. Some athletes, following the recommendations of health experts, choose ornithine – an 'offspring' of arginine and one step closer in the metabolic pathway towards the creation of growth hormone – as a substitute. As it does not participate in so many reactions as arginine it has been reported to be almost twice as effective at stimulating growth-hormone release. Should you suffer from herpes, one highly undesirable effect of arginine is that it may encourage a recurrence of the lesions. Ornithine, though, has no such effect and is certainly the preferred supplement under such circumstances.

Experts suggest that you take a maximum of 6000 mg (6 grams) each of arginine (or ornithine) and lysine, along with 200 mg of B6 and 500 mg of B3. Since growth-hormone release occurs during the night (sleep being another condition for secretion), the best time to take these supplements is just before bedtime and with plenty of water. It should also be taken on an empty stomach. This is because growth hormone also stimulates insulin production. Insulin is a hormone which scavenges for, and then hoards, all the available nutrients it can find (sugars, fats, amino acids, and so on), then stores them inside cells. Should you eat immediately before going to bed, the action of insulin may cause you to put on weight instead of increasing your energy levels.

Summary

Nutritional supplements can be effective in helping to increase your levels of sexual energy. The relevant nutrients are:

- the catabolic amino acids: methionine, taurine, cysteine, asparagine, and glutamic acid
- carnitine for its ability to release energy from the intra-cellular factories known as the mitochondria
- arginine/ornithine and lysine as growth-hormone releasers for increasing the body's metabolic rate and thereby releasing extra energy.

Chapter 8
Oiling Your Lovemaking

Massage can be a luxurious and sensuous part of lovemaking. However, just imagine rubbing the back and limbs of your partner in smooth, penetrating movements without the benefit of massage oil. Oil is a vital component of massage, eliminating friction and enabling your fingers and palms to glide effortlessly over your partner's skin. During lovemaking, the body produces its own massage oil to ease the friction of sexual contact. Without it sex is almost impossible. The source of this lubricating substance, the problems that may interfere with its secretion, and the steps you can take to put things right are what this chapter is about.

Angela is a bright 33-year-old with a flourishing career in a city firm of accountants. She has been married for three years to Henry, a journalist. She came for nutritional counselling after becoming convinced that she was undergoing the menopause.

Calmly and openly she described how making love with Henry had become increasingly difficult during the past six months or so. Basically, during lovemaking and despite her feelings of arousal, her vagina remained dry. Through this lack of lubrication, sexual contact created a painful, burning sensation and she developed a rash that she compared laughingly to a carpet burn. The fact that she was also experiencing uncommonly heavy and painful periods suggested to her the twin symptoms of menopause. Although there are known cases of the menopause occurring this early in life, and although Angela's symptoms led her, quite understandably, to suppose that it had indeed struck her, it seemed highly unlikely that with her active lifestyle and general state of good health this was really the problem. Her doctor examined her, found her in other respects fit and well, and suggested she embark on a programme of hormone treatment. Before agreeing to it, she decided to seek an alternative (in all senses of the word) opinion and came for nutritional counselling.

The first thing she was told was that a dry vagina is a relatively common problem for many females well below the average age for menopause. It might be caused by physical or emotional stress, bad eating habits, environmental pollution, cigarette smoke, alcohol, tea, coffee, cystitis, infection, and perhaps even artificial sex lubricants and other sex aids. Happily it is also a problem that can be resolved. In Angela's case, with careful and patient self-treatment the symptoms faded in a matter of weeks along with her fears of the menopause. She now reports that she is able to make love with her husband freely with no recurrence of the dryness and soreness.

So how was Angela's recovery effected? The first thing was to explain to her a little of the biochemistry involved in vaginal lubrication, and that's what we're going to do now.

Taking to the Tightrope

In lovemaking, the lubricants in the vagina are secreted by the intervention of the parasympathetic nervous system. This is the response that calms the body, generating soothing alpha waves and ensuring that its counterpart, the adrenalin-releasing sympathetic nervous system, doesn't dominate to an unhealthy degree. It is the parasympathetic nervous system that also pumps blood into the penis and clitoris, causing their erection. The importance of the parasympathetic nervous system to lubrication immediately gives us a clue as to what may go wrong. For if the female is suffering from excessive stress, especially if that stress is sustained over a period of time, then the sympathetic nervous system – the stress response – will effectively override the parasympathetic. In the same way that a man may not get an erection when under stress, so a woman's vagina might be prevented from secreting lubricants. This again underlines the tightrope-walk-like balance the body must sustain during sex, this trembling, vertiginous walk between excitation and relaxation. Too much or too little of one or the other overbalances the body's metabolism and it plunges to disaster.

On the other hand, when that balance is maintained, and the sympathetic nervous system fires normally, it causes a particular set of membranes lining the vagina wall just inside the labia to release a sticky substance with a consistency similar to saliva, and it is this that acts as the lubricant.

Understanding the composition of these so-called mucus membranes is the key to discovering the cause of Angela's soreness, dryness, and burning. Let's look at them a little more closely. In common with the walls of every cell and organelle in the body, mucus membranes are made primarily of fatty-based substances called phosphatides or phospholipids. These trident-shaped molecules are composed of two 'prongs' of fatty acids with a third made from a phosphate molecule. It is this phosphate molecule that gives the membrane its most important structural characteristic.

To see just how important the phosphate molecule is, try comparing a phosphatide with its close relative, the triglyceride. Unlike the phosphatide all three of a triglyceride's prongs are made of fatty acids. Non-polar and water resistant, the fatty acids give the triglycerides a tendency to cluster in large clumps and can pose a danger to your health. On the other hand, in a phosphatide, the agglomerating tendency of the two fatty acids is balanced by the polarity of the phosphate, which would like nothing better than to push itself away from all its neighbouring phosphate molecules.

It is these contradictory forces that forge the membrane. While the tendency of the fatty acids is to link up clumps of separate phosphatide molecules together, the phosphate's efforts to push itself away stretches the clumps out into thin diaphanous sheets. At the same time, while the fatty acids shy away from water, the phosphate molecule is water soluble, taking to it like a duck. To protect themselves, therefore, from the surrounding watery environment of the lymph fluids and cytoplasm, the fatty acids draw to them a second 'sheet' of phosphatides. This creates a molecular sandwich in which the filling is the four fatty acids and the 'bread' above and below the two layers of phosphates. This is what we know as the cell membrane. The different chemical properties of the fatty acids and the phosphate allow certain nutrients through the wall, while, rejecting others, they maintain electrical potential by balancing the concentrations between sodium ions outside and potassium ions inside. Let's now look a little more closely at the fatty acids in the membrane, for it is these that hold the key to the lubricating action of the mucus membrane.

Fat in the Middle

You may remember that fatty acids are measured on a sliding scale of biochemical reactivity. Those at the bottom are inert, their forbidding molecular shells as resistant to the occurrence of chemical reactions as the bodice of a Victorian spinster. As triglycerides, at best they insulate the body against the cold; at worst they accumulate in the blood vessels causing high blood pressure, atherosclerosis, and other circulatory problems. As components of phosphatides in the membranes, their role is essentially one of structural support: the herringbone of the aforementioned bodice.

Our attention turns then to those fatty acids at the other end of the scale, the super-polyunsaturates. With numerous spaces in their molecular shells – called double bonds – they are the most chemically reactive substances in the body and thus indispensable for the millions of reactions which they cause and in which they participate. Sitting between the outer phosphate and the inner saturate they are the most important single components of the cell membrane. Each double bond on the polyunsaturate causes it to kink – the more double bonds the greater the number of kinks – so that some resemble the zig-zagging outline of a saw tooth. The fact that each unsaturate is kinked in this way means that they will not pack very closely together with unsaturates from adjoining phosphatides. This creates extra space and in turn means that the cell membrane is more fluid.

The Regulators

Despite the way in which the unsaturates are so vulnerable to damage and their almost promiscuous tendency to react with other substances when they shouldn't, they paradoxically assume formidably powerful regulatory roles. And by creating certain kinds of phosphatide they determine how efficiently mucus is secreted.

The most important of these mucus-generating phosphatides is a variety called lecithin. As a regulator it prevents cholesterol from being deposited on the artery walls and it breaks apart agglomerating fat molecules. This is known as emulsification and it prevents the fat in our blood from rising to our head and shoulders like the oil in a jar of French dressing. You might see lecithin as an ingredient in certain processed foods for this same quality. Lecithin also helps the liver to detoxify poisons, as well as increasing resistance to disease by strengthening the immune system. In the cell membrane it conveys electromagnetic impulses – the prime mover of life – from the energy-producing organelles. You must be sure that it is fresh as it oxidises very quickly.

Most importantly for our purposes, though, lecithin is the parent molecule of a substance called acetycholine. We've already met acetycholine in its role as an inhibitory neurotransmitter. Its calming effects on the brain and in the nervous system are known to be immensely important in helping to enhance the sensual experience and enjoyment of sex. In addition to this, however, a number of researchers, including Durk Pearson and Sandy Shaw, have discovered that it is acetylcholine that causes the membranes within the vagina to release lubricating moisture from their mucus-containing cell tracts.

So what can go wrong? What was it that caused Angela so much pain and distress that she was driven to conclude she was entering the menopause? Simply, while the essential polyunsaturates which make up lecithin are almost alchemically reactive, they are more fragile than a rice-paper spinnaker. Let's see why. Then, having got the measure of the dangers posed to the body's lecithin, we can devise an action plan to ensure that the problems which bedevilled Angela will never arise.

Enemies of the People

We have already encountered some of the dangers posed by free radicals. These, you may remember, are molecules with an unpaired electron. In their headlong search for electrons with which to 'mate', they rob other molecules of their own paired electrons. In pillaging an electron from another molecule, this second molecule will then be compelled to find a substitute electron from a third; it will itself become a free radical. Such a cycle often repeats itself 50,000 times, and sometimes up to 300,000 times, before the body's natural free-radical quenching enzymes step in to halt it.

When the oxidising cycle is adequately controlled by the enzymes, such as in the energy-releasing furnaces of the mitochondria and in the conversion of external stimuli to nerve impulses, free radicals perform vital functions for the health of the body. When it gets out of hand, however, free-radical activity robs the membrane of its fluidity and flexibility (free-radical cross-linkage, after all, is the cause of wrinkling in the skin as we age) and destroy its ability to absorb nutrients and dispose of waste products.

It may also damage the chromosome molecules of the cell. Chromosomes, also known as DNA, are the blueprints of life from which all body structures are made. If the blueprint is altered then those structures which depend on it will be built incorrectly. This alteration may simply lead to membranes which work inefficiently; it may lead to loss of membrane integrity and greater susceptibility to infection. Some researchers believe it may even lead directly to cancer.

However great the consequences prove to be, one thing is certain: the oxidative damage that excess free-radical activity causes is especially prevalent in the hormone-responsive areas of sexual organs such as the lining of the vagina. The extreme vulnerability of fatty acids to such damage means that in some cases the mucous membranes might simply be too badly affected to cause lubrication. Furthermore, if tissue is not repaired as quickly as it should be thanks to the damage caused to the chromosomes, the vaginal wall may itself start to thin.

The next question is: how widespread is excess free-radical activity? Disturbingly, there is mounting evidence to suggest that it is starting to run riot in our bodies. And considering that environmental toxicity (a major source of excess free radicals) on a global scale is now one of humanity's greatest concerns, this is not surprising. Numerous researchers and health writers point out that the success with which we tackle the problems of free-radicals will, during the next two decades, come to be seen as being as important to health as the discovery of the germ theory was in mastering illness. In other words, the idea of free-radical damage is no crackpot, fringe theory. It is an issue that poses the most immediate and undeniable threat to our health.

So how do you safeguard yourself against such problems? The first thing to do, whether you already suffer from a dry vagina during lovemaking or if you simply want to ensure that you never do, is increase your intake of the mucus-generating lecithin. Happily this is widely available in a pleasant-tasting granular form which you can sprinkle on salads, muesli, soups, or desserts. Alternatively you may consider taking a supplement called choline which is, in effect, a concentrated version of lecithin and also widely available.

If you do decide to begin supplementing your diet with these phosphatides, it is also important to complement them with a selection of anti-oxidant (free-radical fighting) nutrients. These include the fat-soluble vitamins A and E, the water-soluble vitamin C, and the mineral selenium. In addition to their individual anti-oxidant abilities, these nutrients are also the main components of the free-radical quenching enzymes superoxide dismutase (SOD) and glutathione peroxidase. And some health experts are now suggesting that by protecting the sensitive mucous membranes these enzymes can actually raise a depressed sex drive. It's up to you how much of each nutrient you take, but suffice it to say that the existing recommended daily amounts are woefully inadequate for most problem cases. To make things a little less complicated, some nutritional-supplement manufacturers have started marketing complexes designed especially to help the body generate these free-radical fighting enzymes.

Wring Out Your Dietary Fat

Your next step should be to cut out as much processed oil as you can from your diet. Many of these oils, such as sunflower and safflower, are our primary sources of certain essential fatty acids: sunflower oil, for example, is rich in the all-important linoleic acid. However, as we discovered in chapter 4, the very act of extracting the oil from the seeds denatures the fatty acids. And when hydrogen is pumped through it to solidify it in order to create margarine, the kinks that are so important for membrane fluidity are 'ironed' out, rendering the fatty acids inert and unable to participate in the acetylcholine-creating process necessary for mucus secretion.

Although we do not recommend cooking with oil at all, it is in all practical circumstances impossible to stop completely. When you do cook with oil, therefore, choose the cold-pressed, extra-virgin varieties of olive oil. It contains primarily mono-unsaturated fatty acids which are less easily damaged by the refining process and will not interfere with the polyunsaturated metabolic pathways which lead to the formation of acetylcholine. As far as cooking with any oil is concerned, here are a few tips. Before heating the oil, sprinkle some water in with it. As the water heats up, it will evaporate, creating a fine mist barrier between the oxygen and the oil while at the same time preventing the oil from becoming quite so hot. This will help to ensure that more of the fatty acids in the oil survive the cooking process intact. Finally, put the food you wish to fry in with your water-and-oil mixture before starting to heat. As soon as you have finished with the oil container, put it in the fridge and preferably in an opaque container. Never reuse the oil you have already fried with.

As for the margarine, use it as little as possible, even if it does claim to be high in polyunsaturates. The denatured polyunsaturates created by hydrogenation are potentially toxic. For an alternative, experts such as the fats and oils authority, Udo Erasmus, recommend you use small quantities of butter. This might sound like heresy in a cholesterol-conscious world and butter is, admittedly, a rich source of saturated fat. However, in small quantities, the fatty acid it contains, butyric acid, can easily be burnt by the body to release energy.

Further Supplements

Most of the preceding suggestions should apply regardless of whether you have problems with the mucous membranes. They should form a standard part of your lifestyle. However, certain supplements can also be used more specifically to target the polyunsaturate-based integrity of those membranes. The first of these is a supplement rich in a fatty acid called gamma linolenic acid. Gamma linolenic acid is used throughout the body for its lubricant qualities, especially in the soft, connective tissue. It oils the mucous membranes around the bones allowing freedom of movement and protecting them from problems such as lumbago, rheumatism, and arthritis. There are very few sources of this lubricant fatty acid in our diets but usually we are able to create it by means of an enzyme from its parent molecule, linolenic acid, a polyunsaturate found in particular in sunflower seeds. However, it is now widely accepted that many of us are deficient in the very enzyme needed to cause that transformation.

The richest source of gamma linolenic acid that we ever feed on is mother's milk. Bearing this in mind it's not surprising that a baby's skin has such a soft, moist, almost creamy texture to it. This same texture should ideally be found in the adult mucous membrane but, without adequate gamma linolenic acid, it may start to coarsen in the same way that our skins coarsen when we are weaned off our mother's milk. Happily, deficiencies can be remedied by taking supplements rich in the essential fatty acids. The best choice would be flax seed oil (sometimes called linseed oil). Borage and blackcurrant are also good choices. If one simply wants gamma linolenic acid, the richest source is a vegetable concentrate called GLA. Do try to take the antioxidant nutrients with it to optimise its effects and protect against rancidity. Some suppliers actually include one or more of these nutrients in with the fatty acid.

As well as improving the sensitivity and receptiveness of the mucous membrane, gamma linolenic acid also produces another regulatory substance called a series 1 prostaglandin. Half hormone, half enzyme, this prostaglandin has been ascribed almost miraculous health-enhancing powers. It reduces water retention, thins the blood, and regulates the body's mineral balance. It is known to mitigate symptoms of pre-menstrual tension, and the cramps, excessive blood loss, and unreasoning irritation and anger of heavy menstrual periods. The fact that Angela, as you may remember, suffered from painful and debilitating periods in conjunction with the dryness of her vagina strongly points to a depletion of gamma linolenic acid.

Flax Fax

Gamma linolenic acid is one of what is known as the omega six varieties of fatty acids. This means that the first double bonds occur at the sixth molecule of the fatty acid's carbon spine. A second, equally important group is the omega three variety. The parent molecule of this group is linolenic acid and its richest source is flax or linseed and its derivative flax oil. Once upon a time flax production thrived thanks to a network of cottage factories. Sadly, since the war especially, this level of production has dwindled almost to nothing in the face of the huge batch presses. Flax oil production is not considered economical by the food conglomerates since, as it is so high in super-polyunsaturated fatty acids, it goes rancid extraordinarily quickly. Consequently, the only widespread use for flax today is in the cricket pavilion with most of its lecithin removed. Better known as linseed oil, it is used to oil cricket bats – a rather sad irony in a chapter on lubrication.

However, even though the unadulterated variety is extremely rare, it is still possible to obtain this lecithin-rich flax oil. The oil itself is available on the continent and can be obtained by mail order. Furthermore, it is comparatively easy to buy linseeds in health-food shops and, with patience, extract the flax oil.

Finally, the other fatty acids of this omega three series are mercifully easier to obtain, both from eating fatty fish such as salmon, trout, and herring and by taking cod liver oil and the now ubiquitous marine-oil supplements. The guidelines for getting the most nutritional value from these foods is the same for any oil-rich food you prepare: keep it cold (preferably refrigerated), keep it in the dark, and supplement your consumption with the antioxidant nutrients, A, E, C, and selenium.

Before we finish, a few words about our old friend histamine (see chapter 6). This, too, appears to assist in the secretion of mucus from the mucous membranes. In this case, nutritionists have discovered that the most effective way of stimulating histamine release in the mucous membranes is with a supplement of niacin (B3), the vitamin responsible for capillary dilation and the skin redness we associate with the sexual flush.

So how were these guidelines applied for Angela? Firstly her average daily diet – including not just food but the way in which it was cooked – was analysed for an excessive consumption of denatured fats. She was understandably taken aback when it was suggested that she replace the low-fat margarine she was using with butter, on the proviso that it was used sparingly. She also admitted that it ran against the grain to fry food with an oil and water mix, let alone placing the food in the oil before heating. She enjoys eating fresh, raw food so it wasn't hard to introduce her to the morning pleasure of fruit and yogurt muesli, sprinkled with two spoonfuls of freshly crushed linseeds. She was also advised to take a supplement of evening primrose oil at breakfast, together with vitamins A, E, and C to optimise its nutritional effects and ward off the possibility of free-radical damage. In the evening she sprinkled lecithin granules on her salads or soups and ate fresh fish at least once a week. In fact, with a superb fishmonger around the corner from their flat selling a wonderful collection of freshly caught fish, she and Henry became enthusiastic sushi cooks. She also took a marine-oil supplement with the meal. Before going to bed she took another evening primrose oil supplement together with a tablet of niacin.

'At first I felt we were going totally overboard by cramming our diets so full of fatty stuff,' said Angela. 'Gradually, though, it started to work its magic. I thought at first it was just taking the niacin that did it, because it gave me a warm, flushing sensation all over. But when I stopped taking niacin, even though the flush wasn't so sudden, there was none of the dryness that I'd been used so. It was great.'

Summary

A dry vagina during lovemaking can be overcome with the help of nutritional supplementation. A blend of the essential polyunsaturated fatty acids are very important. These should include:

- gamma linolenic acid
- the omega 3 series fatty acids such as that found in marine oils and flax oil
- lecithin
- a complex of nutrients to guard against the fatty acids' extreme vulnerability to free-radical-generated oxidation, namely vitamins A, C, E, and selenium.

Chapter 9
Conceiving Immaculately

We're now going to look at some of the problems that you might encounter when attempting to conceive a child with your partner. Although these problems, such as low sperm count, infertility, and miscarriage, don't interfere directly with the act and enjoyment of lovemaking, which is admittedly what this book is first and foremost about, sex is, after all, the means of reproduction. Even in these times of recreation for recreation's sake, good sex is not always an end in itself and at some point in their relationship most couples will decide to have children. Many say afterwards that the lovemaking during their efforts to conceive was happier and gave a greater sense of fulfilment than at any other time.

Sadly, though, many couples have their hopes and expectations dashed. To be told by a doctor that you are unable to conceive, for whatever reason, or to suffer the tragedy of a miscarriage, can impose terrible strains on even the most stable of relationships; more so if, as is sometimes the case, the hope and prospect of a child is the anchor that prevents that couple from drifting apart. In an effort to show you how to relieve some of these traumas if they effect you, this chapter will pinpoint the major metabolic pathways brought into play for conception and highlight those nutrients which play the prominent roles. Let's begin then by looking at the thorny issue of low sperm count.

The Seeds of Fertility

As far as the media is concerned, the nineties are going to be the decade when the baby comes of age. The late eighties have already seen a boom in baby films: *Three Men and a Baby, Look Who's Talking, Raising Arizona,* and *Parenthood,* to name a few. Meanwhile, in slick advertisements for products as diverse as Volkswagen cars and life-assurance policies, the thrusting, jetset executive bachelor of the eighties is reborn as a sympathetic, caring parent more concerned with looking after his kids while the wife goes out to work. If these images really do reflect a trend in society rather than an adman's fantasies, then it's a cause for celebration. At the same time, though, it only hammers home the irony that Western man is probably less capable of conceiving a child with his partner than at any time in history.

At the turn of the century, the average, healthy, adult-male sperm count was in the region of 100 million per cubic centimetre of semen. Now, as we accelerate towards the twenty-first century, that amount has declined startlingly to an average of only 25 million. This might still sound a lot, but you must remember that the attrition rate for sperm as they battle their way through the uterus to fertilise the woman's egg is truly awesome. 5 million is much too close for comfort to the cut-off level at which doctors certify the male as infertile. And more and more men seem to be falling beneath that cut-off figure. So what could possibly have caused this dramatic decline? Let's see.

Once again the spectre of environmental toxicity raises its head above the parapet. Like the mucous membranes of a woman's hormone-responsive sexual tract (see chapter 8), the membranes of a man's testes, seminal vesicles, and prostate gland are rich in essential polyunsaturates. Vulnerability to the free-radicals which damage the membrane phosphatides – such as those contained in carbon monoxide and cigarette smoke – can cause the tissue to repair and regenerate itself inadequately, leading in turn to a withering of the sexual organs and a decline in sperm and semen production. Since these pollutants are also high in heavy metals, they antagonise minerals crucial to health, causing the body to dump them. Particularly at risk is the trace element zinc which, as we'll see, is one of the most important of all nutrients for sexual health.

Another, widely recognised cause of low sperm count is stress. As we've seen, sustained stress causes the body's sympathetic nervous system, the fight-or-flight response, to flood the organism with its excitory catecholamine neurotransmitters such as adrenalin and noradrenalin, as well as the shorter-lived opiate-type substances, the endorphins. In short bursts, these chemicals are important for triggering secretion from the hypothalamus of an aphrodisiac called luteinising-hormone-releasing hormone (LHRH for short). It is this hormone which, as its name suggests, causes the release of luteinising hormone, the chemical responsible for triggering formation within the testes of sperm. However, the effect of longer-term stress is to deplete and suppress production of LHRH and in turn cut the sperm production.

A third factor in the loss of sperm is nutritional. Semen and sperm analysis reveals a concentration of nutrients far above that contained in the body's plasma (plasma is the blood fluid and is taken as the average measurement for the body). These nutrients include several free amino acids (that is, not part of larger protein structures), prostaglandins, calcium, magnesium, sulphur, potassium, B complex, C, and fructose. In chapter 1 we examined at length the difficulty of obtaining a truly balanced diet from the nutrients on offer in modern processed foods. No one, for example, is entirely sure how the hormones and antibiotics used on livestock to encourage growth and protect from infection affect the human hormone system; and mineral shortages are an especially pressing threat to health with today's intensive use of soil phosphates and nitrates together with the mineral-stripping effects of acid rain, which leach important minerals such as calcium, magnesium, and zinc.

Of course, many cases of low sperm count result from genetic abnormalities and certain diseases which we can do nothing about. However, many more can be attributed to one or more of the above factors. If you remember back to the sales manager, Dave, whom we met in the vitality foundation course, his life was choc-a-block with almost every imaginable cause of low sperm count. However, help is at hand. Orthomolecular nutritionists now feel that the problem of low sperm count can, in many cases, be alleviated by providing those nutrients which, for whatever of the above reasons, may be lacking. So let's see which nutrients they are and how they help.

Raising the Count

In 1926, a research programme into the composition of semen

revealed the presence of two amines (chemical derivatives of amino acids) called spermadine and spermine. It is these two substances, the programme discovered, which give semen its characteristic odour. However, it wasn't until the mid-sixties that a link was established between them and sperm production. This link was discovered by a series of tests conducted on the hormone-dependent sexual membranes of men who had undergone vasectomies and on women habitually using the contraceptive pill which was by then widely available. Among the results was a surprise finding which pointed to consistently lower levels of spermadine and spermine within those groups than from fertile men and women outside it.

What the researchers wanted to know was which came first: did the loss of fertility caused respectively by the vasectomy and the pill depress the levels of these two amines, or did the depression of amine levels lead to a loss of fertility? To find out, the research programme was extended to cover victims of low sperm count: men, in other words, who were naturally infertile rather than having had an operation to make them so. The results confirmed the researchers' suspicions for, sure enough, the spermadine and spermine levels in these men were identical to the previous two groups. If low spermadine and spermine levels was the key to infertility, then it seemed possible that, by raising those levels, the low sperm count in the men from the third group could actually be raised. Subsequent work has proved this to be true.

Health experts have found that spermadine and spermine levels can be raised by administering supplements of their parent molecule amino acid, arginine. Together with its B3, B6, folic acid, and magnesium co-factors, arginine is converted progressively to ornithine, putrescine, spermadine, and finally spermine. The maximum recommended daily dose of arginine for achieving this conversion is 8 grams split up throughout the day with meals. However, the presence of one other amino acid, methionine, is essential for assisting the conversion process and should always be included in a formula for raising sperm count.

Does this formula – this blend of arginine, methionine, and co-factors – actually work? In her marvellous book, *Ageless Ageing*, Leslie Kenton reports on one particularly promising recent study conducted on 42 men each of whom suffered from low sperm count. Once they were given arginine and its co-factors, the sperm count of every man doubled soon after the start of the trials. Even better, their sperm motility – the ability of the sperm to move and thus progress their way towards the unfertilised egg – also increased dramatically. To confirm the potency of arginine, when it was removed the subjects' sperm counts dropped back to the levels prior to the start of the tests, then rose once more when arginine was readministered.

Think Zinc

Zinc is another nutrient which is indispensable for sperm motility. Whenever you look at complex protein structures in the body you will find zinc. Together with vitamin C it acts like a tensile molecular cement, giving flexibility to structures such as collagen (skin), myosin (muscle), and lung tissue. Zinc's role in sperm production and motility is very similar to these other roles, since it is intricately bound into the keratin protein molecule which makes up the tail of each spermatozoa and helps to give that tail its characteristic whiplash action. It is this action which, obeying Newton's third law that every action has an equal and opposite reaction, impulses the sperm forward and upward towards the egg. Removing adequate levels of zinc from the keratin tail would be like using a paper streamer for a bullwhip instead of plaited strips of lacquered leather. In short, the sperm's movements would be much less vigorous and, moving more slowly, time would run out on it before it had run the gauntlet of the uterus.

Zinc loss is quite common for a number of reasons. One is the mineral depletion caused by the zealous overuse of fertilisers, which we've looked at quite enough. Another is the act of ejaculation. Zinc is heavily concentrated in the prostate gland and secreted in large amounts with the semen. Some estimates suggest that you can lose as much zinc in a single emission as the entire recommended daily amount. This is probably overstating the case, but zinc loss is still considerable, more so if you, or your partner, are sexually active.

Another cause of zinc loss is smoking. The Tobacco Advisory Council, that august body of philanthropists whose only interest is to state the facts about smoking (ignoring that it is, in fact, the tobacco industry's public relations lobbying arm) often asserts, in its war with the anti-smoking lobby, that nicotine inhalation among non-smokers is very low. No doubt this is true. But focusing on nicotine is really only a devious method of drawing public attention away from other, less palatable facts about tobacco. One of these is that tobacco smoke is one of the richest sources of cadmium. And, measure for measure, cadmium is the most lethal metabolic poison known to man. The cadmium contained in cigarette smoke oxidises vitamin C and antagonises zinc from the lung tissue. Such a loss of crucial nutrients contributes to the stiffening and coarsening of lung tissue, the loss of moisture, and a decline in oxygen-gathering ability which is collectively called emphysema.

The human body has no adequate means of getting rid of cadmium. Non-smokers breathe in around 0.2 mcg of cadmium (which is bad enough), while moderate 20-a-day smokers inhale 16 mcg. While the lungs are the worst-hit organs, once the cadmium gains access to the blood stream it will antagonise zinc wherever it finds it. Not surprisingly, the sperm-zinc level of smokers has been found to be conspicuously less than that of non-smokers. However, non-smokers have no cause to be smug since passive smoking is now such a widely publicised health threat. Meanwhile environmental cadmium levels increase daily from the burning of waste products such as tyres, bin liners, and plastic containers.

A supplement of zinc to counteract these problems, then, makes enormous sense. Some suppliers now provide a useful mix of zinc and vitamin C in a single tablet, which makes a powerful defence against cadmium and its sibling heavy-metal hooligans.

Super Sulphur

One other mineral which is also intimately bound up with the creation and motility of sperm is sulphur. Having written at length about the ills of environmental pollution, praising the virtues of sulphur might seem a little odd. Sulphurous coal is, after all, one of the prime causes of the ecological disasters in Eastern Europe only now coming to light with the dismantling of the old cold-war frontiers. Closer to home, sulphur dioxide is one of the most dangerous emissions from our own power stations. Dispersed in vast clouds over the European continent, and mixing with airborne water vapour, it forms sulphuric acid and falls as acid rain. One in four trees in the Black Forest have died as a result. We are not immune to its effects, though, since the same acid denudes our soil of minerals.

However, despite this, organic sulphur is of enormous importance to the internal workings of the body. It helps to transport elements such as selenium and zinc, promotes supple skin and muscles, attacks and quenches free-radical attack, and encourages the production of protein. And, it is vitally important for the formation of healthy sperm. It helps to bind together the helix-shaped amino acid chains of sperm protein, providing in appearance what can best be compared with the steps of a spiral staircase which link the handrail with the central pillar. Without sulphur, most protein structures would fall prey much more easily to the free-radicals and simply fall apart.

The body uses up around 850 mg of sulphur every day from sources such as eggs, onions, and garlic. Yet even eggs, our richest dietary source of the nutrient, contain only around 65 mg each. To compensate, nature has provided us with a group of three amino acids which, in addition to the standard atoms of carbon, hydrogen, oxygen, and nitrogen, also come equipped with extra atoms of sulphur. These aminos are methionine, taurine, and cysteine, the last of which carries in 1 gram almost three times the amount of sulphur – 180 mg – that you would find in an egg. As well as being the most concentrated form, cysteine is also one of the most easily assimilated. Many nutritionists recommend cysteine as a valuable source of sulphur, and if you wish to take it to assist with sperm formation try 250 mg a day together with co-factors B3, B6, folic acid, and C.

Nutritional Foundations

The fact that there are so many amino acids, minerals, and vitamins employed individually in the creation of sperm means that you would probably benefit from supplements which provided a complex of all of them. It would certainly prove a sound base on which to build the more specific therapies we've just looked at. You could perhaps try a multi-vitamin, multi-mineral supplement together with the complete amino-acid formulation we met in Chapter 3.

It would be wise to take some form of polyunsaturated oils such as flax oil, borage oil, pumpkin seed oil, or concentrated GLA. As well as helping to improve the health of the membranes in the reproductive tract, the ability of gamma linolenic acid to form prostaglandin E1 is very important. This is because, when the prostaglandin in the semen contacts the uterus lining, it causes tiny, rapid contractions and these help to carry the sperm towards the egg. Bearing in mind the extreme biochemical sensitivity of the reproductive tract, the antioxidant nutrients A, E, C, and selenium would also help. Finally, in applying any therapy for raising sperm count it is important to follow the stress-management techniques we examined in the vitality foundation course. You can take all the nutritional supplements in the world, but if your lifestyle is hectic, unfulfilling, and stressful the chances are that you will continue to suffer from the problem you are using the supplements to alleviate.

To Have and to Hold

Assuming that the male partner is able to raise his sperm count with these nutritional and stress-management techniques, what if the woman is unable to conceive? Like her partner, she may have genetic reasons for this inability, which no one can do anything to overcome. However, the failure of some pregnancies is caused simply by the same combination of stress, environmental pollution, and nutritional imbalances as low sperm count, and these are factors which we decidedly can do something to change.

In a woman's body, a successful conception needs the presence of two very special hormones. One is luteinising hormone, which we have encountered already in connection with spermatogenesis. Luteinising hormone serves a somewhat similar function here in that it promotes ovulation, the formation of the ovum or the female germ seed. The other important hormone is called follicle-stimulating hormone and this is responsible for the growth and development of the ovaries. Clearly, unless the ovaries are fully formed and healthy, then no matter how high the sperm count and how tenacious the sperm are in reaching the eggs, fertilisation will simply not occur. These two hormones, like all proteins, are composed of long chains of amino acids. If, for whatever reason (stress, poor digestion, inadequate diet), you are not obtaining all the amino acids and co-factors you need from your food, then luteinising hormone and follicle-stimulating hormone production will be impeded and you will have difficulty conceiving.

Of course, the most natural way for you to obtain these nutrients is from your diet. If necessary change your eating habits and get rid of those aspects of your lifestyle which might cause problems (see chapters 2-4 for tips). As you do, though, a course of the amino-acid complex, together with a multi-vitamin, multi-mineral supplement, will be an excellent way of helping to raise your hormone levels. As far as individual supplements are concerned, one amino acid that is of special value is the sulphur-based cysteine. And, as with all nutritional measures concerned with the hormone-sensitive reproductive tracts, it is important to include a full complement of the antioxidant nutrients to ensure the health and integrity of the cell membranes.

Finally, even after conceiving, some women are threatened with miscarriage due to the imbalance of a hormone called progesterone. This works like a metabolic clock, letting the body know when it's time to go into contractions. Too little of this hormone may terminate the pregnancy, while too much could prolong it beyond its natural term. Interestingly, the most important substance in the formation of progesterone is the fatty-acid derivative, cholesterol. What this means is that expectant mothers should not attempt to cut fatty foods completely out of their diets, as is sometimes tempting. Instead, as well as eating those foods, supplement them with a daily capsule of marine oils. These will help to mobilise cholesterol by creating carrier structures called high-density lipoproteins. Instead of allowing the cholesterol to build up where it is not wanted in the blood vessels and tissue, that ferry it where it is needed or alternatively dump it from the body altogether.

The assistance that these nutrients can give is amply demonstrated by the case of Gina, a publishing firm director. She had already suffered two miscarriages and, when she once again found herself pregnant, she came for nutritional counselling in an attempt to protect herself from another tragedy. Treatment took the form of a high-potency combination of many nutrients, including cysteine, vitamins A, E, C, and B complex, and essential polyunsaturates, as well as multi-vitamin, multi-mineral and complete amino-acid blends. Gina saw her pregnancy through to its natural term and delivered a healthy, happy baby boy.

Summary

Nutritional supplements are important metabolic tools in the efforts of couples to conceive successfully.

For helping to raise sperm count the following nutrients are essential:

- arginine as the precursor of spermine and spermadine
- the sulphur-based aminos methionine, taurine, and cysteine
- zinc and vitamin C
- co-factors A, B3, B6, folic acid, and magnesium.

To assist with ovulation you need a broad formulation of nutrients, including antioxidants and polyunsaturated fatty acids.

Chapter 10
Fine Tuning Your Sexuality

Some readers are probably lucky enough not to have suffered from any of the problems we've looked at so far, but would nevertheless like to discover if there are any nutrients they can take to improve their already satisfactory sexual responses. Happily, many of the supplements we've met in conjunction with rectifying certain sexual disabilities are equally effective in helping simply to 'hone' the experience of lovemaking, ensuring that it is prolonged and its sensations intensified. That's why, in this chapter, we're going to look at some supplements you can use to enhance your lovemaking rather than actually alleviate any difficulties. Some of the nutritional supplements we'll meet have already appeared elsewhere in the book. However, the cyclic nature of the metabolic pathways is such that individual nutrients are used many times over and for a variety of different reactions.

Zinc

Discuss with the average bar-stool philosopher the possibility of using vitamins or minerals as aids for sexual performance and the chances are that, amid knowing winks and painful *double entendres*, he'll tell you that zinc is what you're looking for. Despite the dubious, beery wisdom, though, there will be more than a germ of truth in his assertion. We've already seen the important role that zinc plays in male and female fertility, participating in spermatogenesis and nurturing the ovaries. But did you know that it has also been found to increase libido and intensify the sensation of orgasm?

In a number of studies conducted since the war, zinc has

been found to play a central role in the development of sexual apparatus. A childhood deficiency of zinc, for example, can seriously impair the growth and development of male and female sexual organs. In adulthood, the same deficiency robs the ovaries and testes of zinc and seriously undermines the sex drive. The consequences of this zinc loss are most graphically shown by its effects on dialysis patients. Very simply, dialysis machines are used on people whose kidneys no longer function to filter their blood of waste products such as uric acid. In filtering the blood, though, the dialysis machine is unable to distinguish between toxic waste and important nutrients such as zinc. Although dialysis patients have long been afflicted by atrophy of the testicles and ovaries and loss of libido, it was only comparatively recently that a connection was made between this and the indiscriminate removal of zinc.

However, dialysis patients are not the only people at risk. Even a marginal zinc deficiency – caused by such common-place factors as smoking, imbalances generated by consuming the produce of intensive farming, and stress – will contribute to loss of libido. Carl Pfeiffer of Princeton's Brain Bio Institute was one of many nutrition researchers to discover that supplementing the diets of those suffering from these problems will actually help to alleviate them.

The case of a young man who came for nutritional counselling complaining of low libido proves the point. His lifestyle conformed very closely to the sort of pattern that can lead to zinc deficiency: he smoked heavily, ate mostly processed, packaged food, and worked in a stressful environment. Furthermore he made love frequently, admitting that there was so little pleasure and physical sensation in the act (ejaculation occurred with almost no sense of orgasmic urgency) that for him it had come to resemble a cold, mechanical exercise. Naturally, it was recommended that he improve his diet, exercise, use stress-management techniques and, if possible, give up smoking. However, the single most important piece of advice was the recommendation that he take a daily dose of zinc together with the key co-factors of vitamins B6 and C. He reported back some time later to say that there had been a terrific surge both in libido and strength of sensation at the moment of orgasm.

Zinc and the Prostate

As well as its affect in increasing libido, zinc also has a major bearing on the health of the prostate gland. Ranging in size from one person to another from that of an olive to a walnut, the prostate gland sits at the base of the bladder. During sex it produces and secretes the mucinous seminal fluid into which is mixed the sperm-carrying semen from the testes and seminal vesicles. The seminal fluid acts primarily as a medium for ferrying the sperm a good deal of the way towards the ovaries, ejaculated as it is by the contractions of the prostate gland muscles into the cervix. Weight for weight there is considerably more zinc concentrated in the prostate gland than in any other body organ, including the testes, and there is no doubting the important role it plays in prostate health.

Some younger readers might be tempted to dismiss prostate disorders as a symptom of ageing, without realising how prevalent prostatitis (inflammation of the prostate) is among men in their twenties and thirties, and worsening with age. Prostatitis can cause discomfort and pain as well as lead to difficulty urinating and the embarrassment of incontinence. The need regularly to get up in the middle of the night to urinate is a common sign of prostatitis and is caused by the swollen gland pressing up against the bladder. As well as causing pain and incontinence, it can also interfere with a healthy sexual appetite and is known to reduce libido.

There are a number of causes of prostatitis, including viral and bacterial infection, but one of the most common is zinc deficiency. In a series of tests conducted at hospitals in Chicago, Dr Irving Cook administered zinc supplementation to groups of young men suffering from the problem. In 70 per cent of the cases not caused by infection, the patients experienced a rapid and complete remission of symptoms, reporting freedom from pain and incontinence and a return of libido.

The importance of zinc is further shown by the case of Andy, an organic farmer from Devon, who came for nutritional counselling some years ago. In his late fifties he had begun to experience a bloated, discomforting sensation in his bladder area, which progressively worsened to an acute stabbing pain and occasional incontinence. He had, at the same time, become impotent which, not unnaturally, he found a cause of great anguish and disappointment. A visit to his doctor produced the diagnosis of acute prostatitis with a recommendation of surgery as the only way of treating it. Even so, the doctor thought, it was unlikely that Andy would regain his potency.

As an organic farmer, Andy is naturally open to the precepts of alternative medicine and he decided to come for nutritional advice. The combination of hair analysis and the application of special zinc-measuring taste tests revealed that his body was abnormally low in zinc. How so? He didn't smoke, was under little stress, and followed a fertiliser-free organic diet. However, it transpired that this diet was the key to his zinc loss. Almost all his vegetables were obtained from his own farm and there was every likelihood that the soil was naturally zinc deficient. Such a deficiency wouldn't have affected his customers since they obtained their vegetables from a variety of sources, hopefully balancing out any abnormalities. For Andy, though, living largely off his own soil, the problem had intensified over many years. The solution was to put him on a supplementation programme of zinc together with the necessary co-factors of vitamins B6 and C to help metabolise it. Andy's symptoms of pain and incontinence disappeared in the space of two months. Better still, his libido returned with a vengeance.

Finally, one other interesting fact about zinc is that a deficiency will cause the apocrine sweat glands of the body to emit a strong body odour. This is hardly the sort of thing to attract a lover.

Other Intensifying Nutrients

Fatty-acid derivatives also act to heighten the sensations of lovemaking, increasing arousal, intensifying the physical sensations, and prolonging orgasm. The most important of these are derived from the two groups of essential fatty acids that we've met several times throughout the course of the book: the omega 6 and omega 3 series fatty acids. These substances effect a more intense sexual response for several reasons and we'll look at each in turn.

First, as the precursors of the phosphatides, lecithin and choline, they are essential for the creation of the neurotransmitter acetylcholine. This has a number of roles in the brain and throughout the body tissue. It is a vital component in the memory processes of the brain, for example, and is also mentioned for its ability to stave off the worst effects of depression. It is also, as we've seen, an important ingredient in the lubrication action of the vagina during sexual arousal, releasing moisture from the hormone-sensitive mucous membranes. In addition to these functions, though, it is now known to be intimately involved in transmitting arousal messages from the hypothalamus to the glands and organs of the body, preparing them for sexual activity, changing the brain-wave patterns, and helping to trigger the release of other, excitory neurotransmitters. In this respect, acetylcholine functions as an aphrodisiac, stimulating both mind and body into a greater sense of preparedness.

Another set of by-products of these essential fatty acids concerns itself much more closely with the body's responses after the initial stimulation has occurred and once lovemaking has begun. These products are the prostaglandins, the short-lived, hormone-like regulatory chemicals. Throughout the body they cause specific reactions then, having served their purpose, are instantly broken down by special enzymes. What interests us is that the prostaglandins, among many other roles within the body, are known to help intensify the sexual response at the moment of orgasm. It is these chemicals that cause the shuddering thrusts of the female abdomen at the moment of orgasm and help to trigger the contractions of the prostate and vas deferens which contribute to male ejaculation.

In fact, women who regularly take gamma linolenic supplements – which are the precursors of the most important of the prostaglandins, E1 – report being able to achieve multiple orgasms. While men are, admittedly, not usually able to orgasm repeatedly within a short duration, tests show that increasing the intake of essential polyunsaturates can speed up the time it takes to recover from one orgasm and ejaculation in preparation for the next. Taking fatty-acid supplements (gamma linolenic acid, marine oils, flax oil, lecithin granules, choline) to stimulate greater lubricity, greater desire, and a more prolonged and deeper orgasm would seem to be an obvious nutritional measure for 'fine tuning' the quality of your lovemaking.

As with any supplementation involving polyunsaturated fatty acids, these nutrients should ideally be accompanied by a complementary dosage of the anti-oxidant vitamins A, E, and C, together with the mineral selenium. As we've seen, these will ward off the dangers of rancidity generated by free radicals, helping to optimise the nutritional value of the fatty acids.

Finally, one other set of nutrients for helping to intensify the physical sensations in the genital areas are our oft-encountered friends niacin and histamine. While niacin causes the capillaries to dilate, bringing about the sexual flush and making the skin more sensitive to the touch, it causes histamine to burst from the mast cells of the penis head and clitoris to trigger orgasm. As we've seen before, an excess of histamine will actually cause premature ejaculation, so it is probably not wise to supplement your diet with its parent molecule, histidine, unless you have great difficulty reaching orgasm. Niacin (or vitamin B3), on the other hand, can be used safely for heightening the sensations and pleasurability of touch – of fondling and stroking and foreplay – as well as making the act of penetration that much more gratifying.

Nutrients for Greater Arousal

While the above ensure a greater intensity of sensation, the following nutrients can help to increase your interest in and enthusiasm for sexual activity. The best nutrient for achieving this is phenylalanine. As the parent molecule of the family of catecholamine neurotransmitters, it produces several substances that are closely linked with sexual arousal. The first two of these are called l-dopa and dopamine. L-dopa is, in fact, used to effect temporary remission from the debilitating muscle spasms and loss of motor-neuron control for sufferers of Parkinson's disease. Its calming, inhibitory effect is not what one would naturally link to the physical and emotional arousal of sex. However, considering that the sexual stimulant, acetylcholine, is known to have a similar soothing effect on the motor neurons, the fact that l-dopa also acts as an aphrodisiac isn't so far fetched.

The next two substances in phenylalanine's metabolic pathway also play important roles in sexual responses. These are two excitory neurotransmitters: the brain stimulant noradrenalin and the body stimulant adrenalin. The effects of these chemicals on triggering the sex response are already well covered earlier in this book. However, there is one other offshoot of the phenylalanine metabolic pathway that we haven't already explored. This is the chemical phenylethylamine (PEA). It is this excitory, hormone-like substance that is thought to trigger the emotional sensations of wild, euphoric, romantic, and sometimes obsessive love. The level of attraction to your partner and thus your level of sexual arousal has been found by scientists to be closely linked with the levels of PEA in the body. In his book *Chemistry of Love*, the researcher Michael Liebowitz suggests that PEA creates a romantic euphoria similar in its effects on the body to amphetamines or LSD.

What Liebowitz is less certain about is whether it is the romantic emotions that cause the production of PEA in the metabolic pathways, or whether it is PEA that triggers the sensations of romantic love. If, however, we look at the secretion of a related chemical such as adrenalin, we see that it causes the fight-or-flight instinct rather than the other way round. By the same token this would seem to suggest that PEA plays a similar role in triggering these romantic emotions. This is confirmed by the fact that when PEA has been injected into rats as part of laboratory tests, their responses of physical agitation and 'vocalising' have been found to be almost identical to similar exhibitions of sexual arousal in rats in their natural habitat. What is certain is that the higher the levels of this chemical in the body, the more intense is the partner's sense of attraction towards his or her lover, the greater is the physical desire, and the stronger is the sense of empathy, the emotional bonding that can sometimes make sex an almost transcendent experience.

Another link between the biochemistry of PEA and adrenalin release has been established with the observation that PEA secretion is often triggered when partners fight with each other. Intense emotional conflict – bickering, shouting, screaming, perhaps even pushing one another around – has long been recognised as an aphrodisiac of sorts, and the possibility that this adrenalin-generated activity in turn induces the secretion of PEA might be the reason. It might also account for the unsavoury fact that a lot of people are turned on by acts of violence.

PEA is also linked with adrenalin in its similarity to a drug. When adrenalin is released, people have been known to get high from the stress that triggers it. PEA can become addictive in the same way. Should the partners part for any length of time, their separation can lead to the sort of anxiety that characterises withdrawal symptoms. Likewise, when the partners are reunited this gives rise to a sudden rush of additional PEA release into the body, creating the overwhelming sensations of joy and euphoria at meeting after so long a separation and greatly intensifying the feelings of love, affection, and desire. One essential guideline to remember if you do decide to take phenylalanine to help stimulate any of these pathways is to be certain of ingesting it with its co-factors, namely the vitamins B complex and C and the mineral magnesium.

Extra Energy Nutrients

One nutrient that we haven't encountered up to now is the mineral iodine. Iodine is such an important component of the metabolic pathways that even the British Ministry of Agriculture, Fisheries and Food – perhaps the most conservative of any of its equivalents throughout the Western world in its estimation of the basic nutritional requirements for health – has set a recommended daily amount. Even so it is only a paltry 140 mcg which, when you consider its undoubted importance and the numerous potential causes of deficiency, is laughable. The body contains approximately 40 mg, of which nearly half is concentrated in one organ, the thyroid gland. Found at the base of the neck, this gland uses iodine to manufacture thyroxin, the hormone that governs the body's so-called basal metabolism rate. This is the speed at which oxygen, carbohydrate, and fat is burned in the body to release the energy for cell growth, reproduction, and repair. A deficiency of this iodine-dependent hormone may lead to dry skin, eczema, loss of vitality and energy, low resistance to disease, and obesity. In cases of extreme deficiency, it has also been linked by some researchers to an underdevelopment of sexual organs and impotence. What concerns us, though, is the role it plays in energy release.

We've already seen the role that the anabolic and catabolic phases of metabolism play in releasing energy. These two cycles are closely linked with the activity of the thyroid gland. The thyroid uses thyroxin rather like the quartermaster at a frontier garrison in the nineteenth century might decide on where and how to distribute the supplies in his care. Imagine for a moment that the garrison – in one of the far-flung corners of the British Empire – has been cut off from civilisation by a prolonged attack from a tribe of natives, inspired to a raging bloodlust by the injustices of colonialism. While the garrison itself is well defended, the greatest threat to the occupants' safety lies in the fact that they have only limited stores of food on which to survive. Their hope is that the food will last longer than the natives' siege. It falls to the quartermaster, then, to ration what food the garrison has with ruthless efficiency. There must be no favouritism. Everyone gets as much as they need and no more. Just enough to survive.

Now, to return to the thyroid gland, it serves a similar role in the body to the garrison's quartermaster. In times of plenty, when there are ample raw materials entering the metabolic pathways, the thyroid secretes thyroxin to raise the basal metabolism rate and thus speed up cell growth, enzyme and hormone production, and the breakdown and disposal of waste products. As a corollary of this activity, a lot of energy is also produced and this powers the muscles, aids mental concentration, and encourages greater stamina. Now picture what happens when the supply of raw materials is reduced. With fewer nutrients available to power the metabolic pathways, the thyroid reduces its secretion of thyroxin to conserve what supplies it has, making them available for consumption only as and when it is absolutely necessary. With less food, the basal metabolism rate slows, growth and reproduction become sluggish, and less energy is released. The resulting feelings of torpor, physical heaviness and bloatedness, and lack of mental clarity are typical of low thyroxin secretion and often occur to people on weight-reduction diets. Perversely, though, the fact that the thyroid's activity has been turned right down means that what little food is eaten is stored instead of burnt so that the resulting weight loss is irritatingly minimal. What does this have to do with good sex?

Quite simply, low thyroxin release is not confined merely to dieters. The fact that iodine is the key component of thyroxin means that any deficiency of the mineral will decrease the levels of this hormone and in turn lower the basal metabolism rate. Borderline cases of iodine deficiency are thought to be quite common. Iodine is, for example, displaced from the body by the antagonising effect of the mineral manganese, a substance that is found in relatively high amounts in tea. If you drink more than five or six cups of the stuff a day, it would be wise to cut down. While iodine depletion may lower your energy levels, supplementing your diet with iodine-rich foods will conversely help to stimulate the thyroid gland into secreting additional thyroxin and thus speed up the basal metabolism rate. This means that you will have higher energy levels and that fat, carbohydrate, and oxygen will be burnt more efficiently, in turn providing greater stamina.

The best source of supplemental iodine is organic kelp. It is often administered in tandem with an amino acid called tyrosine. Tyrosine is, in fact, one transformation along the metabolic pathway from its parent amino, phenylalanine. Nutritional experts often recommend this amino acid in phenylalanine's place, however, to ensure that subsequent transformations occur more smoothly. Rather than continuing through other transformations to create the stimulatory substances we've already encountered (adrenalin, l-dopa, and PEA among them), tyrosine is used directly in the thyroid gland to combine with iodine and produce thyroxin. The blend of tyrosine and kelp, together with the important co-factors of B6 and C, stimulate your body into metabolising your food more efficiently and thereby increasing your sexual energy.

The E Plan

Another, supposedly effective, nutrient is vitamin E, a substance often turned to by middle-aged men fearful of losing their potency. Sadly, it's now realised that vitamin E is not the aphrodisiac and sexually potentiating substance that people once thought. Its eminence is probably due to the fact that it is concentrated in the lipid (fat-based) cell membranes of the sexual organs.

This is not to demean it, though. As we've seen, it is enormously important for helping to optimise the effects of other nutrients, in particular the fatty acids. If it does affect your sexual response directly it is through its role as the protector of the walls of the mitochondria, the miniature furnaces inside the cells. By ensuring that fats are burnt efficiently and released as energy it probably complements the action of other, energy-raising nutrients such as iodine and carnitine.

We've now seen what these nutrients can do in theory. In chapter 12 we will look at them in practice.

Summary

If you already enjoy good lovemaking but want to make it even better, certain nutrients can help you to do this, make the sensations more intense. These are:

- zinc, B3, B6, folic acid, and histidine, which make the sensations more intense
- phenylalanine, methionine, zinc, B3, B6, and C, which generate extra libido
- a catabolic amino formulation (methionine, taurine, cysteine, asparagine, and glutamic acid), iodine, arginine and lysine, which provide more energy
- essential fatty-acid supplements (gla, marine oils, and lecithin) and the antioxidant nutrients A, C, E, and selenium, to complete the picture.

Chapter 11
Sex and Herbalism

There's no doubt that so-called conventional medicine no longer carries the weight and authority among the public at large that it did say 20 or 30 years ago. This is not to denigrate conventional medicine. Its advances in medical treatment have been phenomenal. In this century we've seen the back of scourges such as beriberi and tuberculosis; we've witnessed amazing advances in surgical techniques to the extent that surgeons are now able to save the lives of babies by operating on them with minute wires while they are still in the womb; we've marvelled at the spectacular growth in the under-standing of cancer and the steadily increasing survival rates from the disease that have resulted. Yet for all this, there is a growing feeling of disenchantment, a perception that health professionals are more concerned with using their undoubted expertise to suppress symptoms rather than remove causes. As a result people are turning in increasing numbers to alternative methods of treatment.

Ironically, one branch of alternative medicine now enjoying an enormous flowering in popularity is the form from which the roots of modern medicine sprang: herbalism. Herbalism is as old as man's eating habits. It's likely that as our hunter-gatherer forebears learnt which plants they could eat and cultivate – probably through a painful, perhaps deadly, process of trial and error – they discovered simultaneously in certain species powerful restorative and healing qualities. Nowadays, numerous apothecaries, health-food shops, and delicatessens offer a wonderfully wide range of different herbs, each one renowned for its health-enhancing powers.

No doubt herbalism is viewed in some quarters as lacking the necessary scientific base to give it credibility. How, the argument goes, can you claim almost miraculous healing powers for these plants when some are even recognised poisons? It's true, herbs haven't been subjected to the same stringent, exhaustive round of tests that every new drug must endure before it is licensed. Yet these herbs have been used over the centuries by countless hundreds of people. Simply by observing their effects on the metabolism, by being sensitive to the effects of one herb, or a particular combination, on an affliction, by noting the way in which certain symptoms can be relieved, a rich body of lore has grown up around them based on one of the central supporting pillars of conventional medicine: the truth observation.

What little research has been conducted into the nature of herbal remedies seems to confirm their health-enhancing potential. Biochemical analysis shows that many of these herbs have, stored within them, powerful, pharmacologically active substances. These include tannins, volatile oils, secretins, balsams, resins, mucillages, glycosides, and organic vegetable acids. Each effect different responses and participate in different reactions deep within the metabolic pathways. They have recognised anti-inflammatory actions, inhibit the fermentation and putrefaction of food, stimulate the pancreatic secretion of essential digestive enzymes, protect the body against viruses, and help to mobilise fats. They are also thought to influence the secretion of certain neurotransmitters – inhibitory and excitory – in ways which are, as yet, not quite understood.

The herbalist's art is particularly concerned with using the properties of the herbs for their peculiar ability to draw out the body's toxins, irritants, bacteria, and other inflammatory waste products of day-to-day metabolic activity. In this way, resistance to illness and infection is increased, the body's eliminative ability raised, and its vitality and vigour improved. As we saw in chapter 5, if your body is unable to dispose of its metabolic waste products such as ammonia, pus, and dead protein, your sexual health may be severely affected. Therefore, since herbalism concentrates squarely on ensuring that the eliminative processes of your body function at peak capacity, it can help to energise your sex drive.

The herbal remedies that help you to do this can be prepared by a number of methods, depending on the nature of the complaint being treated and your choice of herbs. These methods include:

Infusion Here the remedy is prepared by steeping the chosen herbs. These are generally lighter materials such as leaves, buds, and flowers, although other materials such as ground or finely powdered root, bark, or fibrous material are also suitable. The vessel you choose to steep the herbs in should be sealed airtight so as to prevent the volatile, efficacious elements from escaping in the steam, and allowed to stand for at least 15 minutes with occasional gentle agitation. Although it can be refrigerated, it is advisable to make up only as much of the infusion as you require for a day.

Inhalation The herbs used in this method are those with the highest volatile oil content, such as chamomile, eucalyptus, pine, aniseed, peppermint, menthol, and camphor. Here the preparation is placed into a bowl of freshly boiled, still steaming water. Position your face close over the bowl, drape a towel or tea-cloth over your head to prevent the steam from dispersing, then inhale the fumes in long, deep draughts. By reacting with the mucous membranes of the lungs, herbs absorbed by this method can relieve nasal congestion, inflammation, and sensitivity, although its effects go far beyond the respiratory tract. It can also relieve depression and anxiety, dissipate stress, and encourage emotional balance.

Poultice This is a herb-laden equivalent of a hot compress. After boiling a pan of water with a selection of chopped herbs, the resultant mixture is placed in a muslin bag then pressed up tight against an affected area of the body. It can be used to draw pus and infectants out from wounds, but it is also superb for clearing the lymphatic system of blockages of dead white blood cells and other material, invigorating organs and glands, and eliminating poisons from the cells.

Salve Here the herbs are ground up into a fine powder then mixed with water to create a paste which is subsequently applied to the skin. The nature of this application makes it useful for applying to locally affected areas such as skin suffering from eczema.

What follows is a list of certain herbs that have been observed to have special bearing on different sexual functions. As we've seen, most sexual problems may have one or more of numerous potential causes. Impotence, for example, may result from emotional instability, stress, nutritional disorders, genetic defects, or deep-seated psychological problems. As with the nutritional remedies we have examined throughout the book, this complexity of causes means that your remedy may not entirely eradicate the problem. None the less, herbal remedies can be used both in their own right and to complement the already powerful nutritional therapies we've met.

Many of the following herbs will be available only from specialist herbal suppliers or apothecaries. In some of the following examples we include certain afflictions such as vaginal infection for which, if the symptoms persist, you should consult a trusted health practitioner. One final word of advice: if you do decide to experiment with herbal remedies, we recommend that you consult a recognised herbalist. By discussing your needs and getting an idea of your general state of health, they will be able to recommend the herbs you need with a far greater degree of accuracy and sagacity than you could aspire to with a cursory reading of this necessarily brief chapter. So, without further ado, let's see which herbs are useful for what.

Frigidity Chickweed, damiana, fenugreek, ginseng, plantain, saffron, sarsaparilla, saw palmetto.

Impotence Damiana, Asiatic ginseng, saw palmetto.

Infertility For women, ovarian dysfunction can be relieved with: helonias root, agnus-castus. Helonias root, blue cohosh, and dong quai have all been found to increase fertility. For men, improved fertility may be effected with: damiana, saw palmetto, oats, sarsaparilla, false unicorn.

Pre-menstrual tension Agnus-castus, helonias root, dong quai, parsley.

Prostate Bee pollen, buchu, chaparall, damiana, echinacea, garlic, ginseng, golden seal, juniper, kelp, parsley, queen of the meadow, saw palmetto, uva ursi.

Sexual desire To increase: damiana, ginseng, licorice, saffron, slippery elm.

To decrease: hops, sage, scullcap, willow.

Sexual vitality Dandelion, gotu kola, locorice, yellow dock.

Vaginal infection Typically, infection is kept at bay thanks to the presence of a 'friendly' colony of bacteria which, by converting glucose in the vaginal cell lining to lactic acid, create a protective acid environment. However, factors such as hormone disruption caused by the Pill, menstruation, meno-pause, or excessive alcohol consumption will disrupt this protective lining leading to extreme discomfort and vaginal infections such as thrush, as well as mucoid discharges and urinary problems such as cystitis. These can be treated together either by infusions or with a douche in salve form of: periwinkle, beth root, marigold, arbor-vitae, myrrh, white pond lily, witch hazel.

Chapter 12
Case Studies

Throughout the book we've seen how people's lovemaking can be improved through the practical application of the different nutritional therapies described. In this chapter we're going to look at some more applications, showing how nutritional supplementation has improved the sex lives of those suffering from a variety of problems. In doing so, we'll show you just how effective these nutrients are and how they can be used successfully in your own life. All of the following are real cases of men and women who, during the last few years, have successfully used the nutritional therapies contained in this book. Only their names have been changed to respect their privacy.

Fraser

'My problem,' said Fraser, taking a deep breath, 'is that I suffer from premature ejaculation.' He sat with his girlfriend, Marianne, in the consulting room, his hands clasped, staring out of the window so as to avoid eye contact. He was asked to describe in more detail what happens. 'Well, obviously, when we go to have sex, even during foreplay, it becomes so sensitive to touch that I know any second I'm going to come and there's nothing I can do to stop it.' He had suffered this problem, he admitted, from his mid-teens onwards. As he spoke, his shoulders tense, his voice a dull monotone, it was apparent that the problem had placed him under a severe emotional strain. He recalled how once, during a slow dance with a girl at a school disco, he had ejaculated in his trousers and how, after a number of abortive attempts to have sex, he had been too scared to approach another girl for fear of the humiliation and stigma which he was sure would result.

He was a highly strung and anxious teenager, he said, and this fear had prevented him from having any satisfactory relationship with a woman for eight years. For all that time he had carried his sense of inadequacy like an invisible burden casting a grey pall over his life. Every woman he met he envisaged despising him, and every man he envied for the fact that he didn't suffer from the problem.

He met Marianne at a party. They got on well and arranged to meet again. 'I wanted to take everything ultra slow,' continued Fraser. 'I knew that if we rushed things and went to bed, say, the first time we went out, it would be a complete disaster, so I tried to be calm and never put myself in a position where we would have to sleep together. One time I'd been given a pool car from work to look after for the weekend and took Marianne into the country for a drive. We got back into town late and I was worrying myself stupid that she'd expect to come back to my place. But she said she had to be up early the next morning so I drove her home feeling very relieved.

'I was so tense and anxious that it should go OK. It was torture for most of the time we were together because I wanted so much to tell her about my problem, but was scared I'd drive her away.'

Finally, late one evening, he realised that he'd allowed himself to be cornered. 'We went out for a meal near my place, stayed late, and missed the last tube. I knew I couldn't pack her off in a taxi without her thinking there was something wrong. I felt like a trapped animal, my mind was racing over what I should do, how I could get out of this.' So, with what felt like a 'lump of lead' in his stomach, they trudged back to his flat. 'We lay down on the bed and kissed and it grew more passionate, then we started to help each other out of our clothes and all the time I was thinking "Is this it? Is it going to be OK this time?"' Then, as they touched each other, he started to experience the familiar, helpless sensations of climax and, in a matter of seconds, he had ejaculated. 'I felt so angry and so ashamed.'

'He just kept on saying, "I'm sorry, I'm really sorry," ' says Marianne. 'I tried to interrupt him and tell him that it didn't matter but he wasn't really listening. Then, finally, he opened up to his problem and to the anxiety that he'd carried with him all this time. I didn't realise. It almost made me want to cry to think of all this crippling fear that he'd carried around repressed inside him.'

Marianne is a firm believer in the effects of nutritional supplementation and brought Fraser for a consultation. From the description of his symptoms it was more than likely that he suffered from excess histamine levels and subsequent tests confirmed this. The key to reducing these levels was to discover what the circumstances were that had caused them. A great deal of nutritional counselling concerns itself with having the patient describe in detail his or her lifestyle – what sort of food they eat, what exercise they do, what sort of stress they are under – together with pointers to their state of health. The more that is revealed by these descriptions, the more clues can be garnered and the more accurately links can be established between cause, effect, and cure.

In Fraser's case, he revealed that he had suffered for many years from constipation. He also confessed that his diet at home had been laden with heavily refined food – cakes, tins, and packets – with very little in the way of fresh and raw vegetables and fruit. Then, once at college, the lifestyle there, the lack of facilities, the pressures of work and socialising, encouraged more of the same and by the time he moved into his own flat eating was, for him, a matter of dropping the contents of two packets into a microwave.

The result of such an inadequate diet was to deprive his gut of the fibre it needed to move the food along, slowing down the transit time dramatically. This meant that food and waste products spent much longer than they should sitting in the gut and, as a consequence, started to putrefy. It was clear that putrefaction was a problem for Fraser since he admitted to suffering from both flatulence and fetid stools, while Marianne admitted that he had body odour, all of which are common symptoms. As we've seen, various putrefactive by-products are released into the blood because of this. One of them is histamine.

Normal cell histamine is produced as and when required by the action of conversion enzymes on its parent molecule, histidine. This conversion acts as a metabolic failsafe, preventing too much histamine from finding its way where it is not wanted. However, no such failsafe operates to prevent histamine finding its way into the blood as a product of putrefaction in the digestive tract. It can enter the mast cells and cause mischief by triggering premature ejaculation. Incidentally, this putrefaction probably helped to account for Fraser's emotional instability, since it also produces rogue neurotransmitters that can interfere with the passage of nerve messages and cause behavioural abnormalities.

Although the excess histamine was one cause of Fraser's problem, it was not the only one. The tension and anxiety generated by his fear of ejaculation were also instrumental. We've seen how the sexual response must balance excitation and relaxation on a wafer-thin fulcrum. Fraser's fear-generated adrenalin surges tipped the balance right over so that his worry about premature ejaculation became a self-fulfilling prophecy. The treatment, therefore, would have to treat both the anxiety and the poor digestion.

First, then, to improve Fraser's digestion and transit time, he was given the complete amino-acid complex to stimulate the production of digestive enzymes. A new diet was also formulated for him. Dispensing altogether with the rubbishy convenience foods, they were replaced with foods high in fibre. For immediate relief, though, he was given a fibre product containing psyllium seed husks, pectin, and vitamin C. As for the diet, every day he was to eat at least two apples plus a salad made from a combination of, amongst other ingredients, chopped cabbage, grated carrot, recently soaked and boiled kidney beans, tomatoes, beanshoots, and mushrooms. All of these vegetables would ideally be organic. Rich in natural enzymes, minerals, and vitamins, high in fibre and eaten prior to any cooked food, this salad would help to purge the gut of unwanted toxins and speed up the transit time. The dressing, meanwhile, was to be made from an unadulterated, cold-pressed oil.

It was also recommended that Fraser follow the meal with an organic yogurt rich in the benign lactobacilli which protect the gut lining from toxins and help to digest vitamins. The same yogurt was also to be part of a breakfast muesli of chopped fruit and crushed linseeds. For a man brought up on the virtues of TV dinners and light, fluffy pastries, he said that the cure seemed almost as bad as the problem . . . at least, until Marianne kicked him.

Along with these dietary procedures for improving digestion, he was given other recommendations for nutritional supplementation. It was suggested, for example, that he take the amino acid methionine, together with the relevant co-factors of vitamin B6 and magnesium, to block the cellular effects of excess histamine. And the stress-management techniques we looked at in chapters 3-5 were also described to him, so that, when applied, they would help him to come to terms with the anxiety caused by the prospect of sex and ejaculation. Finally, it was made clear that these measures constituted no instant, miracle cure. They were all part of a programme to which he would have to dedicate himself for weeks, even months. After all, the nutritional deficiencies that had caused the problem had built up over many years and it was unfeasible to expect them to be overcome immediately.

Having established this set of comprehensive guidelines, Fraser and Marianne left to put them into practice. They never visited again but Marianne did write almost a year later. 'Everything is fine,' she wrote. 'It did take a while for things to sort themselves out and the programme was inconvenient at times to administer. There was also the problem of building up trust between us and convincing Fraser that it didn't matter to me if he came at the wrong time. It's a progressive thing and slowly it's started to work its magic and now Fraser makes love to me beautifully.'

Ian

In contrast to the happy, healthy sexual relationship now seemingly being enjoyed by Fraser and Marianne, that between Ian and Fenella started off well then seemed to sink into a trough at which point they decided to come for nutritional counselling. They have been married for nearly two years and during that time had, by their own admission, very good, vigorous sex. They enjoyed experimenting both with new positions – gleaned from every source from *The Kama Sutra* to *She* magazine – and with fresh locations. Things might not have reached the level of Woody Allen's *Everything You Ever Wanted to Know About Sex but were Afraid to Ask* wherein the Italian mod's wife's frigidity only thaws when the two are in highly public places (shops, restaurants), but, none the less, the more public the situation, the more they seemed to enjoy it. 'There wasn't anything exhibitionist about it, really,' says Fenella, 'and we weren't out to offend anyone. It was just the luxury of unfamiliarity. Lovemaking on a hillside or in the sea gives it an added dimension, an urgency.'

'Unfortunately,' says Ian, 'I reached a point where I felt as if I'd burnt myself out. I can't remember when it happened, whether it happened suddenly or just slowly dawned, but I simply lost that important sense of urgency. I didn't feel under any great need to make love any more and when we did have sex I had almost to shake myself mentally to arouse my interest. Then I got tired more easily, didn't find it so pleasurable. It was doubly bad because Fenella was still getting off on it as much as before and she still expected me to show the same commitment. She couldn't understand it some nights when I simply wasn't interested and turned over and went to sleep. Eventually we were going for a week or more without making love, which, believe me, for our marriage is not very good going.'

Fenella was convinced that Ian was tiring of the relationship, that the novelty of their being together had worn off. This might have been true but for the fact that Ian was getting just as lackadaisical in his job as a copywriter. 'I just couldn't concentrate, found it impossible to stop my mind from wondering. Inevitably I started to miss deadlines which just made the pressure worse. Eventually I was walking around like a zombie in a fog. I was like the proverbial athlete hitting the wall.' Ian went to his doctor who, after a lengthy analysis and a blood test, could find nothing wrong. He suggested vaguely that Ian might be suffering from post-viral syndrome, recommended plenty of rest, and prescribed a vitamin supplement. 'I thought, "Thanks a lot, mate, you're a great help, you are."' Then a friend suggested nutritional counselling. Ian thought he had nothing to lose and made an appointment.

To complement the vitamins his doctor had prescribed, Ian was advised firstly to take a supplement of glutamine. This, you may remember, flushes the brain of the toxin ammonia which can easily build up if the waste disposal mechanisms are not working as well as they should. In addition to eradicating ammonia, glutamine can also be used by the body as a brain fuel, contributing to increased concentration and alertness, together with a calmer, clearer thought process. The glutamine was to be taken with the complementary folic acid, vitamin B6, and vitamin C. In addition to this, Ian was also given a small programme of nutritional supplementation consisting of: phenylalanine to stimulate the catecholamine-producing metabolic pathways and thereby raise his interest and enthusiasm for life; carnitine to help liberate extra energy for stamina by transporting the fatty acids to cell mitochondria for burning; and arginine and iodine to provide extra energy and thyroxin for the muscles to cope with the demands on them from physical activity, especially sex.

The results of this supplementation were quite dramatic. 'I immediately felt more alert and more sensitive to what was going on around me,' says Ian. 'The best way of describing it is to compare it to playing a piece of music first on a clapped-out old tape recorder then on a CD. The reproduction on the tape recorder – muffled, distorted – was the way my mind had been working for weeks. The reproduction on the CD player – sparklingly clear, textured, and precise – was how I felt afterwards.'

Gradually his enthusiasm returned together with his sense of vigour, and playfulness. 'I took Fenella out to dinner and as soon as we sat down, seeing her sitting there across the table from me, I couldn't wait to get her home. We played footsie under the table all through the meal and we just had to leave before the sweet because neither of us could stand it any longer.'

Amanda

Amanda is in her late thirties. She is, she admits, scared of old age and, following her divorce, has dated a succession of men much younger than herself. 'My last boyfriend and I recently split up,' she says, sitting in the slanting sunlight of a late afternoon in August. 'There were other reasons, I'm sure, but the one that sticks in my craw is that he said I'm useless in bed. Sure, if he's going to use that as a reason then I don't want to have anything to do with him anyway. But the trouble is, I do have difficulty making love sometimes.' Amanda went on to explain the tension she experiences, the lack of energy or desire, the dryness of her vagina during penetration. Setting aside, for the moment, the importance of lovemaking with a partner who is sensitive to your needs and can support you when you experience difficulties – rather than someone who would rather desert you at the first sign of trouble – what sort of nutritional measures could be devised for Amanda to help her over her problems?

Firstly, for the dryness, she was given a set of guidelines for fatty-acid supplementation. She was to eliminate as much as possible the processed oils in foods such as margarines and bulk-produced vegetable oils. She was to sprinkle lecithin granules and freshly crunched linseeds on her food and take supplements both of gamma linolenic acid and marine oils. She was to eat as much fresh fish as she could – a minimum of once a week – while cutting down on the saturate-containing red meats. Then, to support this, she was to take a complement of anti-oxidant nutrients, vitamins A, E, C, and the mineral selenium.

Then, to enhance Amanda's feelings of arousal and desire, it was suggested she take a supplement of phenylalanine – the precursor of, amongst others, the aphrodisiac neurotransmitter, phenylethylamine (PEA) – together with zinc, niacin (B3), and B6 to heighten sensations of pleasurability. And finally, to help release extra energy, she was given a supplement of carnitine, together with a blend of the catabolic aminos methionine, cystein, and taurine. The catabolic aminos were to be taken specifically in the late afternoon or early evening to coincide with and stimulate, the catabolic (energy-releasing) cycle of her body.

Eschewing her former preferences, Amanda subsequently met, and married, an older divorcee whose sympathy and sensitivity to her problems were of enormous assistance in helping her to overcome her problems. However, she is convinced that the nutrients helped her and continues to take them today.

Angela

Somewhat similar symptoms affected Angela, although for markedly different reasons. A pretty, vivacious 27-year-old cello player, Angela found herself suffering from loss of energy and dryness of the vagina. However, these problems were only corollaries of the main reason for her coming for nutritional counselling. Angela was anorexic. As a teenager she had been abnormally sensitive about her appearance and, determined as she was to succeed at everything, she dieted stringently to achieve the slim appearance she felt she wanted. Anorexia, however, is characterised by an inability to perceive yourself as you really are and, while others might remark on your slimness, even gauntness, noticing the angular cheekbones, prominent joints, and thin limbs, you see only the ugly fat that you are desperate to get rid of. The enforced dieting and, if you are bulimic, the self-induced vomiting, quite understandably cause catastrophic nutritional imbalances. This loss of raw-material nutrients, particularly to the neurotransmitters, only contributes to clouded self-perception and exaggerated mood swings.

Angela came for counselling on the advice of a friend in a voluntary anorexia aid centre who convinced her that, since many nutrients were low or non-calorie, there would be no problem about triggering weight gain if she took them. Once she started talking about her problems it was as if a floodgate had been opened. She was remarkably forthright and perceptive in admitting how destructive anorexia is, yet unable to rid herself of the compulsion to diet. It had become very bad recently as she had started seeing a new boyfriend with whom she had fallen in love. Her determination to please him meant that she wanted more than ever to lose weight. However, perversely, the less she ate, the more weight she put on. The weight gain was marginal, admittedly, but it infuriated her. At the same time she experienced a dramatic loss of energy. In bed with her boyfriend, she felt languid and unresponsive, and once even went to sleep in the middle of their lovemaking.

There is an interesting reason for this. The body's anabolic/catabolic cycle acts, as we've seen, according to the prevailing metabolic environment. The fact that Angela had deprived herself of food to such an extent meant that the anabolic cycle – the process of building up and storing – had been brought predominantly into play. Since the raw-material nutrients so essential for growth and repair were at such meagre levels, the body was compelled to store and hoard everything it could find. And, to make sure that none was lost, the catabolic – tearing apart – cycle was reduced. This was an act of the body attempting to save its own life and accounts for the minor weight gain experienced by Angela. It also explains her loss of energy.

Since it is the catabolic cycle that releases energy, the loss of catabolic activity so that food could be hoarded deprived her body of stamina and energy, and led in turn to Angela's overpowering feelings of languor. In order to raise her energy levels, therefore, it would be important to administer the catabolic formula. However, to do so without helping Angela's overall metabolism would have been grossly irresponsible. First, then, she was given the amino acid complete blend together with the aminos glutamine and phenylalanine to assist in promoting mental and emotional clarity. She was also administered a cross-section of important co-factor minerals and vitamins.

It was only when she had been following this programme for two or three weeks that she was moved onto the catabolic formulation and she quickly experienced a surge in her energy levels. She is now undergoing special therapy to help her overcome her anorexia. In the meantime, she and her boyfriend enjoy energetic sex. They should be married by the time you read this. You may wonder what the relevance of this story is for you. Simply, you don't have to be anorexic to experience an anabolically generated loss of energy. If, for example, you decide to embark on a severe slimming diet then it may well have the same effect of energy loss and sexual languor. (Being lodged in the anabolic phase during dieting, incidentally, is one reason why many people put on so much weight when they stop dieting; the body simply stores all the extra food as if in a siege mentality. The catabolic formula is therefore a useful dieting aid.)

Gerry

Gerry's problem is that he has been unable to ejaculate for getting on for a year. When making love to his girlfriend he finds it impossible to orgasm no matter how long the intercourse lasts. 'At first it was a bit of a joke between us,' he says. 'My girlfriend, Naomi, would say, "For God's sake, can't you fake it?" and we both had a good laugh.' It's starting to be a problem now. Quite apart from the fact that it gives me very little gratification, it causes Naomi quite a lot of soreness. We try to get around this by using lubricant jellies but, frankly, she must get a bit bored hanging around waiting for me to come. We do experiment with foreplay and that has had some success but obviously it's nowhere near as satisfying.'

Testing showed, not surprisingly, a low level of blood histidine and a marginally deficient level of zinc. Accordingly, Gerry was given a programme of niacin supplementation to diffuse the capillaries and trigger the sexual flush that releases histamine from the mast cells, together with additional histidine to raise the mast cell concentration of histamine in preparation. He was also given a zinc supplement to take together with its co-factor in the prostate, vitamin B6. He was to take the niacin no more than 15 minutes before sex, a recommendation that he followed religiously and, after a fortnight, was delighted to report a dramatic lowering of the time it took him to achieve orgasm and ejaculation. 'It still takes quite a long time – which is fine by me – but the important thing now is that I can experience the satisfaction and fulfilment.'

Linda

Linda's problem is not dissimilar to Gerry's. 'I don't think I have ever had an orgasm when making love to a man. Mind, I've made it a practice of never telling them. They have such vulnerable egos. I'd sooner fake it than go through all the recriminations and navel-gazing that results from a man discovering that he can't make you come.' Linda recently started going steady with Graham and thought: 'Hell, if we're going to spend the rest of our lives together then I'm going to be open with him about this. I want him to make me orgasm when we make love, otherwise how can it be making love?' When she told him, Graham was a model of understanding and together they started looking for ways of helping Linda to achieve orgasm. Their investigations led them to the beneficial uses of nutritional supplementation.

'I sorted out a whole bunch of stuff to take: pills and capsules, you know. There was zinc, niacin, histidine, evening primrose oil (this last, as the precursor of prostaglandin El, assists in the contractions of orgasm) 'and marine oil. It was pretty funny us trying to compare my responses from one night to the next, but after a few weeks they were really doing their job. Yeah, Graham's pretty pleased about it, that's for sure.'

Klaus

Klaus is a businessman who has married comparatively late in life to Simone, a young woman 15 years his junior. 'We both want children desperately', he says. 'I've spent the last 20 years or so travelling from one country to another, negotiating export deals, arranging contracts, living in one faceless hotel after another. I've never put any roots down. I want to create something special with Simone. I really want children.' The problem is, continues Klaus, that after almost a year of trying to conceive they have so far not been able to do so.

'It put our marriage under a lot of strain,' says Simone. 'This baby was a way of atoning for what he saw as a lot of wasted time in his past, and when I didn't get pregnant he blamed me. He was convinced that it was my fault – which was pretty hurtful – and made me go for tests. However, they all proved that I was perfectly healthy and quite capable of conceiving. So Klaus was tested and it showed that his sperm count was very low indeed. It was a great blow to him but a salutary experience too, I hope. He can be very arrogant.'

Klaus visited a number of specialists who, while by no means encouraging optimism, said that in some circumstances it was possible to raise the sperm count. Stress management was an especially important means of treatment and Klaus would have to learn how to avert the anxiety-generating pressures of his job. He was also to get rid of some of the flab that had accumulated as the result of untold numbers of business lunches by exercising for half an hour every day. Finally, a specialist recommended that he also try nutritional counselling. 'We're quite desperate,' repeated Klaus. 'I'm not getting any younger. We want to have children. Very badly. Can you help us?'

First, it was made clear that nutritional supplementation can give no more of a cast-iron guarantee than any other means of treatment. His low sperm count might, for instance, have been genetically inherited, which would mean that there was nothing anyone could do to help him. Once it was clear that supplementation was no panacea, a comprehensive nutritional programme was devised for him that addressed as many of the possible nutritional deficiencies as possible. He was given the amino acid arginine (the precursor of spermine and spermadine) and the sulphur-based aminos methionine, taurine, and cysteine, together with co-factors zinc, vitamin B6, and magnesium, all to assist with spermatogenesis and increase sperm motility. He was also given a blend of fatty-acid supplements – gamma linolenic acid, marine oils, lecithin – to promote the integrity of the hormone-responsive membranes of the testes, together with the important anti-oxidant co-factors, vitamins A, E, and C, and selenium.

At the time of writing, it's too soon after starting to administer the supplementation programme to know for certain what the results will be, whether Klaus's sperm count will indeed rise sufficiently for Simone to be able to conceive. However, with the combined stress management, exercise, and nutritional therapies, his specialists have detected a considerable increase in both sperm count and motility. The prognosis, in other words, is good.

These stories illustrate just how effective nutritional supplementation can be when targeted on the relevant metabolic pathways. What they also show, by and large, is how important it is to have an understanding, sensitive partner. The good sex nutrition programme, after all, is about assisting the interaction between two responsive people, not about showing an individual how to hone their sexual athleticism regardless of their partner's feelings. As we've said before, nutritional supplementation doesn't bring results overnight. For these measures to work their magic, and to ensure that you can continue to take them for as long as necessary, you must have a partner who has as much confidence in their powers as you do yourself.

Chapter 13
The Foods of Love

Up to now we've concentrated almost entirely on using nutritional supplements as tools to help energise your sex drive. In an ideal world, of course, we would be able to obtain all of these nutrients from our food rather than as supplements. However, thanks to the threat of nutritional insufficiency (and quite possibly even deficiency) brought about by a combination of the factors we examined in chapter 1, obtaining from your food all the nutrients needed to supply the body's sexually related metabolic pathways is not always easy. As it is, much of our food is pathetically limited in the important nutrients it has to offer us. This is why, therefore, we have recommended supplementing your diet with the food's constituent nutrients.

In this chapter, however, we step back from scrutinising the individual, good-sex nutritional supplements, to look instead at the richest food sources of these nutrients. Some of these foods are renowned for their aphrodisiac qualities and this may well be because they are nature's most concentrated sources of nutrients such as zinc, phenylalanine, and histidine. The following lists, therefore, chart those foods with the highest levels of each of the key nutrients we've met during the last dozen chapters. From these you may be able to formulate your own good-sex menus, creating delicious meals for you and your loved one (or intended loved one), which will help to stimulate and excite the relevant metabolic pathways.

HISTIDINE Assists in lubrication of the vagina wall, increases physical intensity of orgasm, and combats frigidity and/or inability to orgasm. Excess may contribute to premature ejaculation.

Per 100 g

Parmesan cheese	1609 mg	Tuna	1599 mg
Pork chop	1412 mg	Dried seaweed	1085 mg
Skinless chicken	963 mg	Dried non-fat milk	951 mg
Skinless turkey	915 mg	Bacon	889 mg
Cheddar cheese	872 mg	Peanuts	748 mg
Whole dry milk	714 mg	Ham	711 mg
Roast beef	676 mg	Skinless duck	620 mg
Cottage cheese	574 mg	Beef liver	524 mg
Lamb	501 mg	Ricotta cheese	459 mg

METHIONINE Combats premature ejaculation and assists phenylalanine in fighting stress and depression and raising energy levels.

Per 100 g

Dried seaweed	1148 mg	Parmesan cheese	1114 mg
Brazil nuts	1014 mg	Dried non-fat milk	881 mg
Sole/flounder	870 mg	Skinless chicken br.	859 mg
Skinless turkey	849 mg	Cod	800 mg
Tuna	799 mg	Salmon	783 mg
Veal cutlets	758 mg	Skinless chicken leg	748 mg
Halibut	731 mg	Herring	709 mg
Pork chop	686 mg	Whole dry milk	660 mg
Skinless duck	635 mg	Mackerel	632 mg
Sardines	615 mg	Egg	576 mg
Red snapper	574 mg	Haddock	568 mg
Trout	557 mg	Shrimp	544 mg
Rabbit	541 mg	Ham	524 mg
Cottage cheese	520 mg	Crab	519 mg
Roast beef	484 mg		

PHENYLALANINE Combats stress and depression, increases libido and raises energy levels.

Per 100 g

Dried seaweed	2778 mg	Parmesan cheese	2234 mg
Dried non-fat milk	1694 mg	Dried peanuts	1467 mg
Veal cutlets	1364 mg	Cheddar cheese	1308 mg
Whole dry milk	1270 mg	Skinless chicken br.	1231 mg

Pistachio nuts	1184 mg	Bacon	1175 mg
Sunflower seeds	1169 mg	Skinless turkey	1164 mg
Lean pork chop	1114 mg	Almonds	1113 mg
Sole/flounder	1110 mg	Chicken leg	1072 mg
Cod	1011 mg	Tuna	1000 mg
Salmon	999 mg	Beef liver	993 mg
Skinless duck	984 mg	Halibut	933 mg
Cottage cheese	931 mg	Herring	906 mg
Roast ham	857 mg	Egg	840 mg
Crab	830 mg	Mackerel	805 mg
Roast beef	802 mg	Rabbit	793 mg

TRYPTOPHAN Food sources of Tryptophan are (in descending order of concentration):

Spirulina, dried seaweed, parmesan cheese, pumpkin seeds, sesame seeds, veal cutlets, lean pork chops, milk, chicken, almonds, sunflower seeds.

SELENIUM Guards against free-radical activity and in particular oxidation of the sensitive membrane tissue of sexual organs.

Per 100 g

Butter	146 mcg	Herring	141 mcg
Brazil nuts	103 mcg	Lobster	65 mcg
Shrimp	59 mcg	Oats	56 mcg
Crab	51 mcg	Oysters	49 mcg
Milk	48 mcg	Cod	43 mcg
Wholemeal bread	40 mcg	Brown rice	39 mcg
Steak	34 mcg	Lamb	30 mcg
Turnips	27 mcg	Orange juice	19 mcg
Beer	19 mcg	Egg yolk	18 mcg
Mushrooms	12 mcg	Chicken	12 mcg
Radishes	4 mcg	Almonds	2 mcg
Kidney beans	2 mcg	Carrots	2 mcg

ZINC Helps to intensify physical sensations and heighten libido, combat frigidity and/or inability to orgasm, and assists with formation and motility of sperm. Food sources of Zinc are: Wheatgerm, corn bran, oysters, popcorn, sesame seeds, pumpkin seeds, cashews, pecans, roast beef, hamburger patty, lamb, milk, cheese.

Per 100 g

Steak	5.5 mg	Lamb chop	5.5 mg
Brazil nuts	4 mg	Beef liver	4 mg
Egg yolk	3.5 mg	Oats	3 mg
Almonds	3 mg	Sardines	3 mg
Chicken	2.5 mg	Hazelnuts	2.5 mg
Anchovies	2 mg	Tuna	2 mg
Haddock	2 mg	Shrimp	1.5 mg
Turnips	1 mg	Parsley	1 mg
Potatoes	1 mg	Carrots	0.5 mg
Milk	0.5 mg	Wholemeal bread	0.5 mg
Grape juice	0.5 mg	Pork chops	0.5 mg
Olive oil	0.5 mg		

ESSENTIAL POLYUNSATURATED FATTY ACIDS May assist with embryo conception and in raising sperm count and motility, and help to lubricate hitherto dry vaginal walls, improve digestion, and combat PMT.

Linoleic acid per 100 g

Safflower oil	73.4 g	Corn oil	57.3 g
Walnuts	35.2 g	Peanut oil	31 g
Sunflower seeds	30 g	Brazil nuts	25 g
Sesame seeds	23.3 g	Pecan nuts	16.9 g
Peanuts	14.2 g	Pistachio	10.2 g
Almonds	9.8 g	Olive oil	8.2 g
Filbert nuts	6.3 g	Bacon	5.6 g
Plain popcorn	3.3 g	Cashew nuts	3.2 g
Avocado	1.7 g	Lamb	1.3 g
Turkey	1.3 g	Pork	1.2 g

Best direct sources of gamma linolenic acid (%)

Borage	24	Algae	15
Blackcurrant*	15–19	Gooseberry	10–12
Evening Primrose Oil	2–9		

*Blackcurrant also contains a natural GLA inhibitor and is not recommended as a source.

Best sources of linolenic acid (%)

Linseeds	49–52	Pumpkin	15
Soya oil	3–9	Walnut oil	<1
Dark green vegetables	<1		

Best source of omega 3 (EPA) fatty acid per 100 g

Anchovy	747 mg	Salmon	633 mg
Herring	606 mg	Mackerel	585 mg
Tuna	337 mg	Halibut	194 mg
Cod	93 mg	Trout	84 mg
Haddock	72 mg	Swordfish	30 mg
Red snapper	19 mg	Sole	10 mg

Vitamin A
Food sources of Vitamin A are:
Liver, carrots, sweet potato, apricots, squash, seaweed, parsley, watercress, mangos, cantaloupes, milk, fish, peaches, papayas, broccoli.

Additional sources of vitamin A as Beta-Carotene include carrots and bell peppers.

Vitamin C
Food sources of Vitamin C are:
Raw guavas, raw sweet peppers, kiwi fruit, raw broccoli, raw parsley, raw cauliflower, raw papayas, raw watercress.

Vitamin E
Food sources of Vitamin E are:
Corn oil, sunflower seeds, safflower oil, wheatgerm, peanut oil, almonds, sesame seeds, pecans, walnuts, olive oil, cashews.

Vitamin B complex
Food source of B complex are:
Wheatgerm, brewers yeast, chorella, and other sea plants.

Chapter 14
Good-Sex Guidelines

Our aim in this chapter is to tie up those loose ends left from previous chapters by giving you advice on how to put the information in this book into practice. In the following pages, therefore, we'll highlight a selection of the nutritional supplements you should be looking out for which can best help to improve your sex life; page 164 carries important precautions to follow when taking these supplements; while if you turn to page 169, you'll see a list of recommended further reading should you want to examine in greater depth individual topics covered here. Finally, on page 167 you'll find a 'ready reckoner' for quick reference to show which nutrient is important for helping to enhance which area of sexual activity.

First, though, we'll address a question that many would-be subscribers to the benefits of nutritional supplementation ask: namely, how do you know for certain that your sexual problem stems from a nutritional imbalance? After reading this book, you may simply want to go out and purchase those supplements which, from the information we've looked at, seems most likely to help you. Alternatively, a nutritional counsellor, after a thorough discussion of your symptoms, may recommend a programme of supplements for you. The arguments in favour of nutritional supplementation are strong and their restorative powers are not in doubt, but some people feel – quite justifiably perhaps – that there is too much trial and error involved here. If you share this view then there are actually a number of tests that you can have performed to assess your body's nutritional status prior to using nutritional supplementation. None are exhaustive in their own right. Some pinpoint certain mineral deficiencies, should they exist, others concentrate on amino-acid levels. None-the-less, they can be a useful means of discovering with a greater degree of certainty which supplements your body needs. So let's look at the most effective and reliable of these.

Amino Acid Testing

The most accurate way of assessing the level of your body's amino-acid profile is with what is known as a quantitative urinary amino-acid screening. Although few nutritional counsellors possess the facilities to perform such tests themselves, many do maintain arrangements with laboratories that are able to carry the tests out for them. In order to perform such a test, the patient must first collect all the urine from a 24-hour period. Since a fraction of all the nutrients circulating in the blood stream is siphoned off by the purifying filter process of the kidneys and subsequently spilled into the urine, this testing is a fairly accurate measure of the body's current nutritional status and is especially suited to measuring the amino-acid pool. Collecting the urine is crucial for the ultimate accuracy of the test, since it covers the body's full metabolic cycle, both the building up, anabolic, phase and the tearing down, catabolic, phase.

Once is has been collected the urine is then centrifuged and subjected to a process called high-pressure liquid chromatography. Here, electrically charged resin molecules are used to highlight the relative concentrations of each of the 22 available amino acids. The readings are then measured against the expected norm. Any shortfall, or indeed excess, can be rectified using the supplementation methods we've looked at. As we say, this method also works for nutrient groups other than amino acids. However, if you are looking solely to judge your body's minerals levels, there are other, cheaper, and probably quicker ways of doing so and we'll look at a selection of them next.

Blood Testing

Although it is often used by medical authorities to determine the levels of minerals in the body, it is recognised that blood testing can present a misleading picture. This is because levels of certain minerals may be more or less concentrated in areas of the body – tissue, glands, bones – other than the blood. Two cases in point are the minerals that have figured predominantly in this book: zinc and iodine. As we've seen, each of these is concentrated heavily in specific, localised areas. Zinc is found in the prostate, iodine in the thyroid. Therefore, even if a blood test were to show that your blood was low in zinc, the unwary observer's interpretation that this problem was necessarily bodywide may not be true. Likewise, when interpreting mineral levels in blood testing it is also crucial to be aware of the relationship of different minerals to each other. A prime example of this is a reading that indicates a high calcium level in your blood. The immediate response would be to feel confident that you have plenty of dietary calcium and that you are therefore probably well protected from problems such as osteoporosis. However, it may in fact mean that, perversely, your body's magnesium levels are low. This is because magnesium helps the body to produce a hormone called calcitonin and it is this that stores the calcium safely and healthily away in the bones. Less magnesium means less calcitonin and the consequence of calcium leaching out from the bones. Ultimately, then, high blood calcium may possibly even indicate that the bones are in an unhealthy state of calcium loss. Although this situation is only hypothetical, it does illustrate the importance of sensitivity to the metabolic fluctuations in your diet.

For the same reasons, blood testing should be treated warily as a means of assessing the degree of heavy-metal toxicity in your body. In Britain recently, the Ministry of Agriculture was forced to reveal that it had allowed foodstuffs heavily laden with lead to be fed to dairy herds for three weeks before taking any action. With characteristic mendacity it has since refused to account for what happened to the lead-laced milk taken from the affected cows. Was this milk knowingly allowed to enter the food chain? And if it did, how are we to trace it? Disturbingly, it is only when a person dies and his or her skeleton is analysed that a picture of the true extent of lead toxicity can be established. This is because, when the body senses the presence of lead, it does its damnedest to stash it as far away as possible from the vulnerable enzyme systems, membrane tissue, cells, and hormones. It does this by stuffing it, and other heavy metals such as the mercury which is thought to leach from fillings, into the comparatively inert structures of the bone. Therefore, even though blood levels may suggest satisfactorily small heavy-metal levels, this testing gives no indication of their concentration in the bones.

One aspect of mineral analysis for which blood testing is ideally suited is assessing iron and copper levels. This is because these two minerals perform their important oxygen-carrying tasks in the blood's haemoglobin cells. Furthermore, since copper antagonises zinc, an elevated copper level may well suggest that the all-important zinc is being dumped from the body to compensate.

All in all, to get much value from blood analysis you need to be sensitive to the causes of different fluctuations and to follow up different signs with the craft and suspicion of a detective. Even so, since blood testing, like urinary analysis, only shows the body's current nutrient status, obtaining an accurate reading can be a bit of a lottery.

Hair Analysis

For assessment of heavy metal toxicity, hair analysis is considered a much more accurate form of testing. In his book *Trace Elements, Hair Analysis and Nutrition*, Richard Passwater describes hair as 'permanently recording past events on your elemental status'. Hair grows at a rate of approximately 6 inches a year. During this time, small quantities of minerals are constantly deposited in the hair stem and their concentrations here are much the same as their levels in the body as a whole. Hair therefore makes a useful indicator of the body's mineral status, not just as it is at that moment in time, but how it has been for the preceding months. As with the other tests, there are certain pitfalls to avoid when interpreting the results of hair analysis, but these are much easier to spot. For example, some shampoos contain the mineral selenium; washing regularly with such preparations would lead to a hair analysis that suggested extraordinary high levels of selenium. Swimming in public baths also interferes with analysis since the high concentrations of copper in the water might give the impression that body levels of copper are similarly high. This in turn could mislead you into supposing that your zinc levels must have been antagonised as a result, causing you to take zinc supplements when it might not be necessary. Finally, bleaching or highlighting the hair denudes it of a broad cross-section of minerals, therefore rendering it unsuitable for hair analysis.

Against these reservations, the one overridingly positive factor in its favour is that, unlike urine or blood analysis, hair doesn't just present a picture of your nutrient status as it is at the moment of testing. Rather, since hair is constantly growing and taking fresh deposits of minerals into its stem as it does so, analysing it can reveal developing nutritional trends stretching back many months. In revealing how your mineral levels have fluctuated during the growth period, it is possible actually to map out the way in which your metabolism responds to the week-in, week-out activities of your life. One further benefit of hair analysis is that it can pick up the presence of heavy-metal toxicity with a far higher degree of accuracy than other tests. This is because the hair used, along with the bones, to store heavy metals as far out of harm's way as possible.

Zinc Testing

One ingenious method devised specifically to appraise approximately the body's zinc levels is available from Nature's Best (see page 170 for address). This test involves simply swilling a specially formulated zinc solution around your mouth. The aftertaste you are left with will very much depend on how high your body's zinc level is. The accuracy of the test is due to the fact that zinc is an important component of our sense of taste. The higher the zinc levels in our taste buds and nasal lining the more pronounced our taste will be. If, on the other hand, the solution leaves no taste after you have swilled with it, then there will be every likelihood that your body will be suffering from a shortage of the element. (It's no surprise that smokers do consistently badly in this zinc test since the cadmium contained in cigarette smoke badly antagonises the zinc. As a rule smokers have a notoriously bad sense of taste.)

Iodine

Iodine testing can be performed very simply in your own home. Simply purchase a bottle of tincture of iodine – which you will find in most chemists and drug stores – then paint a two-inch square strip on the inside of your thigh before retiring to bed. When you wake, simply examine the area. If the patch of iodine is still visible then your body's iodine levels are at least satisfactory. If, on the other hand, the patch has disappeared, it could well be that the skin has wholly absorbed the iodine to make up for a shortfall elsewhere in the body. Probably the most unreliable aspect of this test is the fact that examining the inside of your thigh is not the first thing you would remember to do when you wake up in the morning.

Urinalysis
There are some new interpretations of this oldest clinical assessment tool that allow indications of a person's ability to digest, absorb and transport nutrients to the cells.

Supplementary Guidelines

Assuming that you have decided to use nutritional supplements, perhaps for the first time, which ones should you choose? Looking at the selection of supplements in even the most modest of health-food shops can be a bewildering experience because of the sheer diversity of brands, formulas, and strengths to choose from. How will you know that the supplement you are picking is going to be the correct one for you? The following are a few simple pointers to guide you when you make your selection.

Amino Acids

1 Complete blend
If you decide you would like to supplement your diet with the complete amino-acid complex, make sure that the supplement you choose contains only amino acids rather than a mixture of amino acids together with what is known as protein powder. Some brands of protein powder – which are products used primarily by athletes and body builders to help create muscle bulk – carry claims from their manufacturers to contain all the essential amino acids. Since amino acids are the building blocks of protein this rather shameless piece of marketing is not, strictly speaking, untrue. However, in the case of these powders, they are bound up in more complex, complete protein forms. This means that when you ingest the powder,

the body will then have to expend energy in secreting enzymes to help break down the protein into its simpler amino-acid raw materials. This defeats the purpose of taking amino acids in the first place. The beauty of free-form amino acids found in reputable complete-blend products is that they are already, in effect, 'pre-digested'. Therefore, they pass straight through the intestinal mucosa without straining the body's digestive system.

Another problem to watch out for when deciding on a complete amino-acid blend is that the separate amino acids are contained in broadly the correct proportions. A good blend should contain 20 of the most important and widely used amino acids mixed in proportions that correspond to those found in chicken eggs. Sometimes, though, manufacturers try to load the blend with the more cheaply produced amino acids such as glycrine. If the blend you find on the health-store shelf doesn't contain a similar percentage mix of amino acids to the following table then look for another:

Alanine	2.5	Leucine	9.0
Arginine	9.0	Lysine	10.0
Aspartic acid	2.0	Methionine	5.0
Cysteine	0.5	Phenylalanine	5.0
Citrulline	1.5	Proline	2.0
Glutamic acid	10.0	Serine	5.0
Glutamine	10.0	Threonine	4.0
Glycine	3.5	Tryptophan	3.0
Histidine	2.0	Taurine	1.0
Isoleucine	6.0	Valine	5.0

Together with a small amount of excipients.

To summarise: ensure that the blend contains only free-form amino acids, no protein or hydrolised protein, and that the constituents are mixed in the above quantities.

2 Individual amino acids

In nature, amino acids have both an 'l' and a 'd' form. What this means is that one is a mirror image of the other. The amino acid supplements you will find on the health-food shelves usually contain the 'l' form since researchers have found it to be considerably more efficacious. Therefore, unless your nutritional counsellor has specifically recommended other-wise, always buy 'l' form. The one exception to this general rule is our friend phenylalanine. Researchers have found that while the 'l' form stimulates the catecholamine-producing metabolic pathway, the 'd' form helps to prolong the existence of the opiate-like pain-killing substances, the endorphins. Consequently, the two have something of a complementary effect. This is why the 'l' and 'd' forms are often sold together in a complex called dl phenylalanine, more commonly known simply as DLPA.

Minerals

It has been established that there are two separate mechanisms for absorbing minerals into the body. One is a complex mechanism for inorganic salts that requires an acid medium to dissolve the salts and amino acids in the cells. The other is with organic amino acid chelates which are absorbed directly without interference. The latter, while expensive, is generally worth the extra cost. Mineral supplements should be taken under the guidance of a nutritional expert, who has access to forms not readily available. However, if on your own, the following include some of the more readily available forms.

Calcium
Calcium ascorbate   A calcium form of vitamin C that is well assimilated.
Calcium aspartate   A well-absorbed amino acid chelate.
Calcium gluconate   A non amino-acid chelated form that is readily absorbed, but must be broken apart and re-combined with amino acids before it can be used.

Copper
Although most forms of copper are easily absorbed, copper amino acid chelate is the preferred form.

Iodine
Seaweeds and kelp are naturally rich and easily absorbed sources of iodine. However, due to pollution, these sources may be contaminated with mercury, cadmium, etc.

Magnesium
Magnesium ascorbate   This form of magnesium is in fact a variety of vitamin C. Consequently it is easily absorbed in the

gut and rapidly transported through the body.

Magnesium aspartate   This is an amino-acid chelate (carried into the body by the hooking action of an amino transport molecule) which is similarly absorbed well in the body.

Magnesium orotate   A form of magnesium whose acidity assists gut absorption.

Magnesium gluconate   A chelated glucose-derived salt which is absorbed well, but requires the body to split it apart and combine it with appropriate amino acids before it can be used.

Selenium

Selenate and/or seleno-methionine   These two varieties of selenium – the first a salt, the second a chelate – should ideally be taken as one to derive maximum effect.

Zinc

Zinc amino-acid chelate   Probably the best way of zinc supplementation.

Zinc citrate   A form of citric acid. Well absorbed and metabolised.

Zinc piccolinate   A form of the easily absorbed piccolinic acid.

Vitamins

Likely as not, the available choice of vitamins will be greater than any other supplement group. The quality is generally high among reputable suppliers, most of which employ stringent quality-control standards.

Precautions

Nothing is completely safe if you take it in sufficiently high quantities but, since the supplements we've looked at in this book are themselves high-potency, natural foods you will need to take amounts well in excess of the recommended daily requirements to experience any sort of adverse effect. Many people, for example, take more than a gram a day of the water-soluble vitamin C when the RDA is a paltry 30 mg (33 times less than a gram). There are, though, certain precautions you should to take and we'll look at these now.

Keep Your Mind on Co-Factoring

In reality this is only reiterating a point we've made all through the book: namely, if you are using nutritional supplementation to relieve a specific disorder, don't fall into the trap of thinking that simply taking the nutrient at the start of the metabolic pathway you wish to affect – for example, histidine for inducing orgasm – will eradicate the problem. All metabolic pathways need the active participation of many co-factor vitamins and minerals for synthesizing enzymes and effecting the conversion of one nutrient to another. If, therefore, you suffered from frigidity or lack of physical sensation during lovemaking, both of which are symptoms of low histidine/histamine, simply taking a histidine supplement would not be a sufficient remedy. On the contrary, it may tax the pool of co-factors in your body, drawing on vitamins and minerals that would otherwise be used elsewhere and consequently possibly even contributing to deficiencies itself. Therefore, even though individual nutrients can be of enormous benefit, we do stress the importance of developing an awareness of the interdependence of raw materials within the metabolic pathways. What this means in practice is to follow those guidelines we set in each chapter. Always include a balance of co-factors with every substrate nutrient you take.

Warnings in Particular Circumstances

Phenylketonuria
Never take any variety of phenylalanine if you suffer from phenylketonuria. This is a genetic inability to manufacture the enzyme that converts phenylalanine to tyrosine, the first stage of its metabolic pathway. Unless converted the amino acid has been known to cause mental retardation in the very young.

MAO Inhibitors
Do not take phenylalanine, tyrosine, or tryptophan if you are taking a monoamine oxidase inhibitor. This is a variety of antidepressant which is prescribed under several different brand names. MAO inhibitors work by blocking the enzyme

Sex, Health and Nutrition

that naturally breaks down neurotransmitters such as adrenalin and serotonin. It is prescribed to relieve depression, anxiety, and stress. If your supplementation of the above aminos coincided with using a MAO inhibitor, there would be potential for an overload of the relevant neurotransmitters leading to a range of mood-related disorders.

Tryptophan
The current controversy about the withdrawal of tryptophan from sale has already been covered in this book.

High Blood Pressure
If you have a history of this problem only take l-phenylalanine, DLPA, tyrosine, or tryptophan under your doctor's guidance.

Herpes and Arginine
Laboratory tests have indicated that arginine can stimulate the resurgence of a latent herpes virus. Although this work is largely theoretical, it is worth substituting ornithine in its place if you have a history of herpes.

Good Sex Ready Reckoner

For quick reference, this chart summarises the different nutritional remedies that we've met throughout the book.

Problem/disorder	Remedy
Anxiety	tryptophan; B3; B6; folic acid: C
Clumsiness	glycine; gamma amino butyric acid (GABA); B6; folic acid; C
Depression/stress	phenylalanine and/or tyrosine; methionine; magnesium; B3; B6; C
Difficulty conceiving	complete amino acid blend; marine oils; cysteine; lecithin; A; B complex; C; E; selenium
Dry vaginal walls	gamma linolenic acid; marine oils; flax oils; lecithin; histidine; A; E; C; selenium
Frigidity and/or inability to orgasm	histidine; B3; B6; zinc
Lack of libido	phenylalanine; B3; B6; folic acid; C; zinc
Lack of physical intensity	histidine; B3; B6; zinc
Lack of libido/ low energy levels	phenylalanine; catabolic nutrients (methionine, cysteine, asparagine, glutamic acid); carnitine; arginine; A; B6; B12; folic acid; C; E
Lack of mental alertness	glutamic acid; B6; folic acid; C
Low sperm count/ low motility	complete amino-acid blend; arginine; cysteine; gamma linolenic acid;

	marine oils; A; B3; B6; folic acid; magnesium; zinc
PMT	gamma linolenic acid; A; B complex; C; E; selenium
Poor digestion	complete amino-acid blend; lecithin; increased polyunsaturate intake; high raw, fresh, food intake; psyllium husk supplement
Premature ejaculation	methionine; calcium; magnesium; complete amino-acid blend; high fibre food; high raw food intake

Further Reading

Ageless Ageing, Kenton, L., Century, London, 1986.
The Amino Revolution, Erdmann, R., Century, London, 1987.
The Bitter Pill, Grant, Dr E., Corgi, London, 1985.
The Chemistry of Life, Rose, S., Penguin, London, 1985.
Fats and Oils, Erasmus, U., Alive, Vancouver, 1986.
Fats, Nutrition and Health, Erdmann, R., Thorsons, London, 1990.
The Healing of Cancer, Lynes, B., Marcus Books, Queensville, 1989.
Life Extension, Pearson, D., Warner, New York, 1980.
Love, Sex and Nutrition, Jensen, Dr B., Avery, New York, 1988.
The Magic of Magnesium, Trimmer, Dr E., Thorsons, London, 1987.
Personality Strength and Psychochemical Energy: How to Increase Your Total Performance, Watson, G., Harper & Row, London, 1979.

Supplement Suppliers

Advanced Nutrition Limited
8 Chilston Road
Tunbridge Wells
England
TN4 9LT
Telephone: 0892 515927

Nature's Best
PO Box 1
Tunbridge Wells
Kent
TN2 3EQ
Telephone: 0892 534143

Index